ULTRA-RIPPED ABS

The Musclebuilder's Body Parts Series

ULTRA- RIPPED ABS

Robert Kennedy

Sterling Publishing Co., Inc. New York

Acknowledgments

The success of this book is not just the work of the author. My first obligation is to the IFBB. Without this organization, headed by Ben Weider, there would be no organized bodybuilding as we know it today. Similarly, without Joseph Weider, bodybuilding would not be as well publicized as it is.

Robert Hernandez, my editor at Sterling Publishing Co., keeps my writing at its best, and often has to put in more effort than I care to admit. My thanks and appreciation for Jim Anderson's artistic creativeness in the design of the book.

To World's and Gold's gyms, both of which have always shown me courtesy and willingness to give me every opportunity to take photographs at their establishments—thank you!

And the photographers who have done so much. Special thanks is due to Steve Douglas, Paula Crane, Art Zeller, Bill Heimanson, Doris Barrilleaux, Chris Lund, Denie Walter, Garry Bartlett, Walt Sorenson, Robert Nailon, Doug White, Al Antuck, Bob Gruskin, John Campos, Jim Marchand, Monty Heron, Tapio Hautala, Bob Flippin, Peter Potter, Edward Hankey, John Balik, Mike Neveaux, Reg Bradford, Wayne Gallasch, Paul Goode, Ken Korentayer, Glenn Low, Lou Parees, Roger Shelley, Bill Reynolds, Russ Warner, Eric Chapman, George Greenwood, Joe Valdez, and my custom photoprocessor, Mike Read.

Edited by Robert Hernandez
Designed by Jim Anderson

Library of Congress Cataloging-in-Publication Data

Kennedy, Robert, 1938–
 Ultra-ripped abs.

 Includes index.
  1. Exercise. 2. Abdomen. 3. Bodybuilding.
I. Title.
GV508.K46 1987   646.7'5   87-10124
ISBN 0-8069-6416-2 (pbk.)

Contents

Introduction

The waistline is the truest indicator of your body's overall condition. If it is well muscled, tight, and devoid of fat, then so is the rest of your body.

Many people believe that the biceps are the most obvious examples of a person's muscularity, but it's the abs that count. When a true bodybuilder is in shape and you ask him or her about their condition, you won't see a flexed arm for the proof. Instead, the bodybuilder will pull up his or her shirt and you'll be treated to an eyeful of finely sculpted, chunky abdominal muscles. That's the real test.

Unfortunately, even in today's fitness-conscious world, we still have millions of men, women, and youths who are hardly aware of their abdominal muscles. Why? Because they are hidden in a sea of adipose—fat. Yet every one of us has ab muscles. True, some may be better developed than others, but underneath that fat we have rows of abdominals waiting to be coaxed to the surface. You could become proud of your small, well-muscled waistline instead of ashamed of its flabby appearance and oversized dimensions.

In this day and age, there are numerous ways to lose that fat midsection, but do they work? What is the truth about diet pills, rubber belts, vibrating-belt machines, and wraps? I'll get to the hearts of those matters in the next chapter. I will also detail the best and healthiest way for you to custom taylor a diet and exercise plan to obtain a dynamic new midsection. Unlikely as it may seem to you now, I know you can do it.

A word of caution: Before undertaking this or any other program of exercise, or change in diet, consult your doctor.

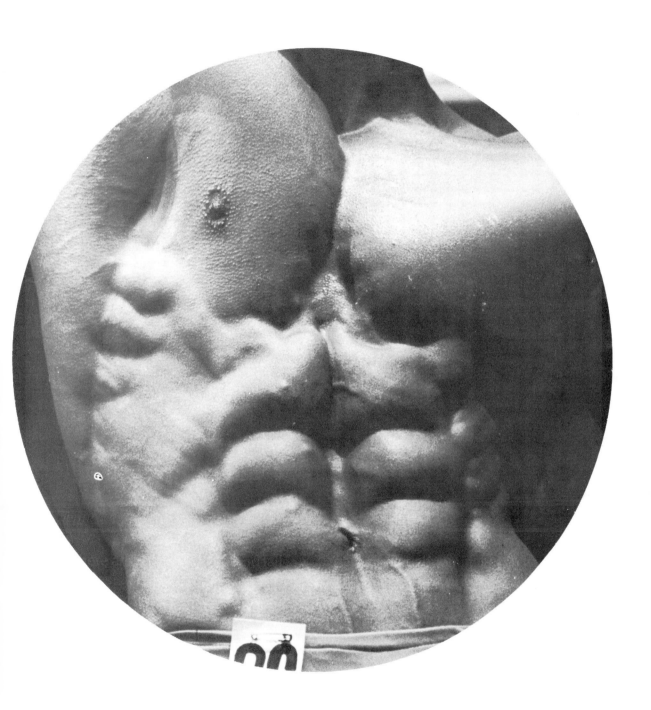

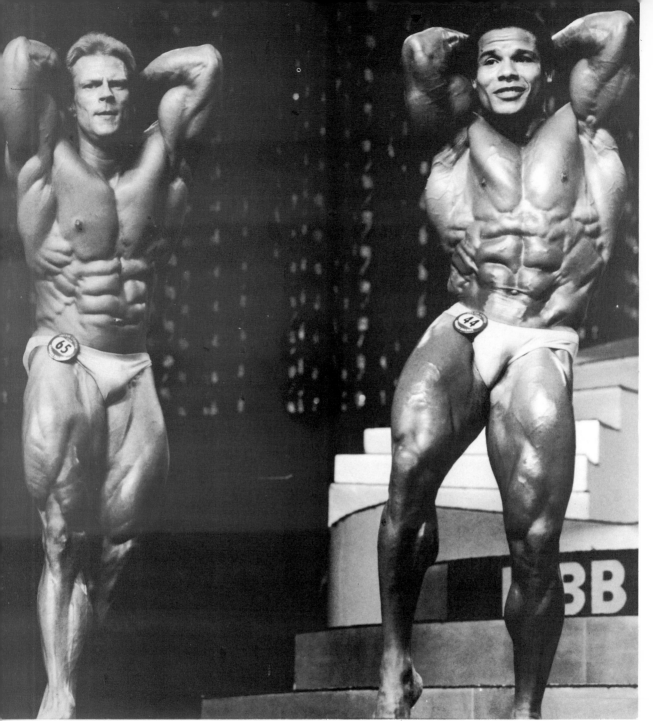

John Hnatyschak and el Shahat Mabrouk

Ask him or her to refer you to someone who can arrange to give you a stress test. Then a judgment can be made about your suitability for performing a strenuous exercise program. Chances are, of course, that your physician will be able to recommend it at once, but it's always advisable to have this checkup. Certainly, people who have a history of health problems, and those who smoke or are over forty years of age, should definitely consult their doctors. Once you've gotten the green light, you can proceed with enthusiasm and confidence.

How long does it take to get a fat-free, well-muscled midsection? That depends on you. Half of your success depends on your persistence. The other half depends on how far out of shape you have allowed your waistline to become!

If you are very overweight, you cannot expect to look perfect by the end of next week. Fat should only be lost at the rate of about two pounds a week. That may not sound like much, but it translates into fifty pounds in six months or one hundred pounds in a year. I have known overweight people who lost ten-to-fifteen pounds in one week but then never succeeded in attaining their goals. Their crazy methods of diet and exercise left them exhausted and almost sick, and they never carried on with their methods to the proper conclusion. Invariably, they quit and gained back all their excess pounds . . . and more.

A sensible diet coupled with an invigorating exercise plan for the abdominals is the quickest, healthiest way to a well-tapered midsection. In this book, you'll find plenty of exercises and routines for developing and trimming the upper, middle, and lower abdominals, including the sides. Discover how such top bodybuilding stars as Mohamed Makkawy, Corinna Everson, Samir Bannout, Rachel McLish, and ten others train their abs into title-winning shape.

Men and women who have nice tight midsections have a renewed confidence. They are proud of their bodies. Follow me through the pages of this book and I'll show you how to make some dramatic changes in your appearance. Now that you've taken the first step, move onward.

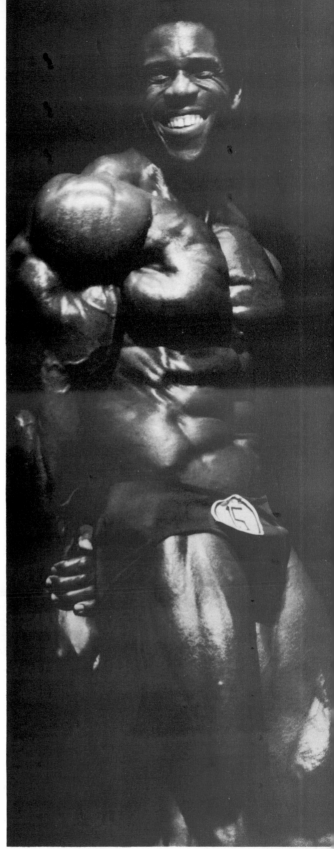

Britain's Bertil Fox

Clare Furr

Myths about the Midsection

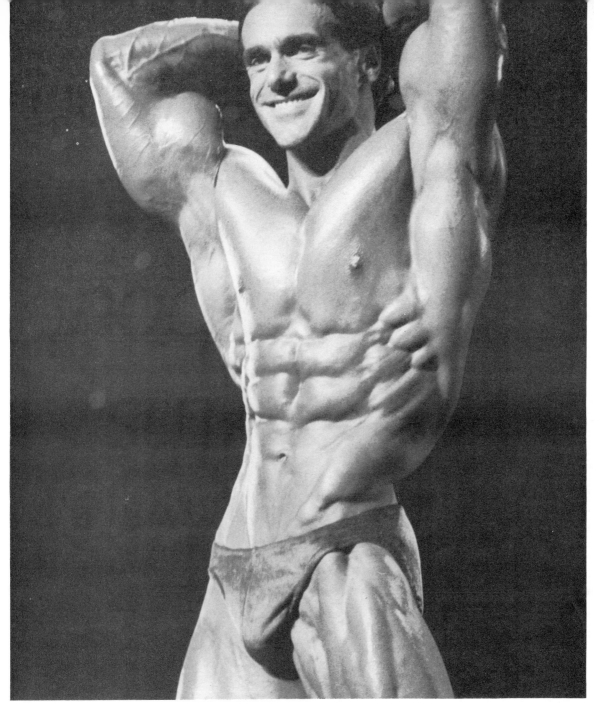

John Terilli

There are so many myths and fallacies about developing a fat-free waistline that people often don't know where to turn for believable advice. Instinctively, we all know that physical activity burns calories and helps us to lose weight. We are also aware that abdominal exercises will firm up the stomach muscles, and that eating fewer calories will bring down our fat percentage. However, we are still looking for a magic pill that will do it all for us effortlessly—and we want it to happen instantly. This world is full of gimmicks

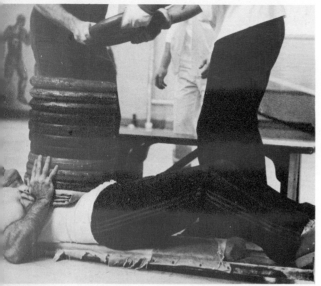

This three-photo sequence shows Howie Dean of Canada performing a sit-up with an incredible 550 pounds!

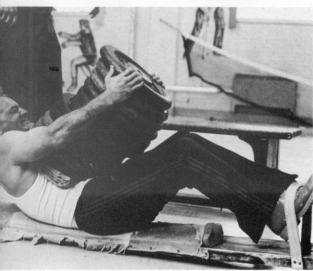

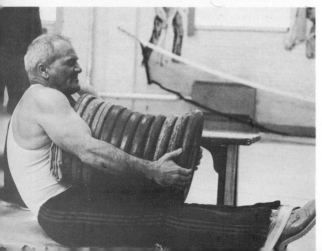

and gismos to give us smaller, better-toned midsections. Some work reasonably well, a few offer only minimal benefits, and others are little short of fraudulent.

Vibrating-Belt Machines

These small, electrically driven machines have a wide vibrating belt that can be placed around your stomach, hips, lower back, or thighs. The shaking movement is like a rough massage, and after five minutes on one of these machines you feel as if you've been through a tough workout. But, in reality, all they do is shake your fat around. Cells can be broken down by these machines and you can feel pretty uncomfortable the next day, if not sick, but the action does not translate into better-looking abdominals. These machines are rarely, if ever, used today, and for good reason—they don't do anything.

Wraps

This is a process in which a part of your body (usually the waistline) is tightly wrapped with a rubberized, elastic wrap to produce an instant weight loss. Creams are used to help the effect. Because the skin cannot breathe, sweating is induced and a small decrease in inches is achieved. However, it all comes back as soon as you stand up, resume your normal activity, and drink fluids. This method is a favorite last-resort treatment of some women who want to be able to fit into a particular piece of clothing for an important function. Invariably, it is only a very temporary solution, and that person doing it is soon bursting at the seams. Body wrapping is also expensive. I do not recommend it.

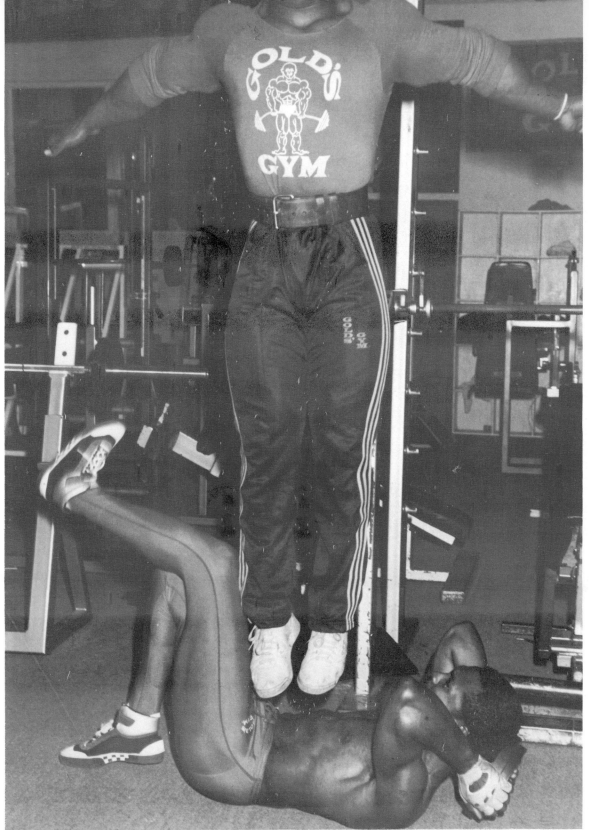

Jerry Bell proves that he has tough abs by allowing Aaron Baker to jump on them. Definitely not recommended!

Diet Pills

There are three types of diet pills which profess to help you lose weight. None of them are recommended unless specifically prescribed by your doctor to correct a medical problem. The first type is supposed to curb your appetite. These could be of some use, at least theoretically, but I've tried them, and so have many other people, and I have never heard anyone say they worked.

The second type of pill possesses an ingredient that revs up your metabolism so that you burn up energy like crazy. The trouble is that you become nervous, highly strung, weak, and shaky after taking these pills. And they're not suited to the bodybuilder's needs because they tend to deplete not only fat cells, but also muscle mass.

Thirdly, there are diuretics, frequently used by bodybuilders who hate to diet. Taking diuretics is a bad idea because not only do they flush out fluid from under the skin (which is good) but they also take water out of the muscle cell itself. They are unhealthy to use because they flush out important minerals from the system and can cause serious health problems. Diuretic users can be spotted at physique contests. They are the ones with flat-looking muscles and drawn faces.

Starvation Diets

If you reduce your food intake too drastically, you will run the risk of putting your body into shock. You literally rob your body of important protein and nutrients that it needs to stay healthy and function normally. It lowers your resistance to illness. When you almost starve yourself, the body gets the message that it may be in for a long period without nutrition. It may then automatically slow down your metabolism and hold on to stored fat supplies. Oddly enough, some people even gain weight on excessively low-calorie diets. It's far better to reduce your caloric intake sensibly and progressively each week or so.

Leg Raises and Sit-Ups

Traditionally, these two exercises have been performed for hundreds of years to develop and tone the abdominal muscles. However, many professional trainers now do not consider them to be the best exercises for the waistline at all. Trainer Vince Gironda said, "Sit-ups and leg raises are not ab movements. They do nothing for the waist area, and could even prove harmful to your back!" (see the chapter entitled, "The 15 Best Abdominal Exercises.")

Spot Reducing

Hardly a day goes by when I am not asked to recommend a good abdominal exercise to reduce excess weight around the middle. The question presupposes that excess fat can be reduced from a specific area by exercising that area. Such is not the case. Spot reducing, as the concept is known, is not a workable solution. Weight-reduction plans affect the whole body. No better proof exists to dispel the theory that concentrating on a specific body part with a particular exercise will develop it than our picture of marine captain Alan Jones who trained daily to be able to perform some 27,003 sit-ups. Study the photograph. The man's not overweight, yet there's hardly an abdominal muscle in sight!

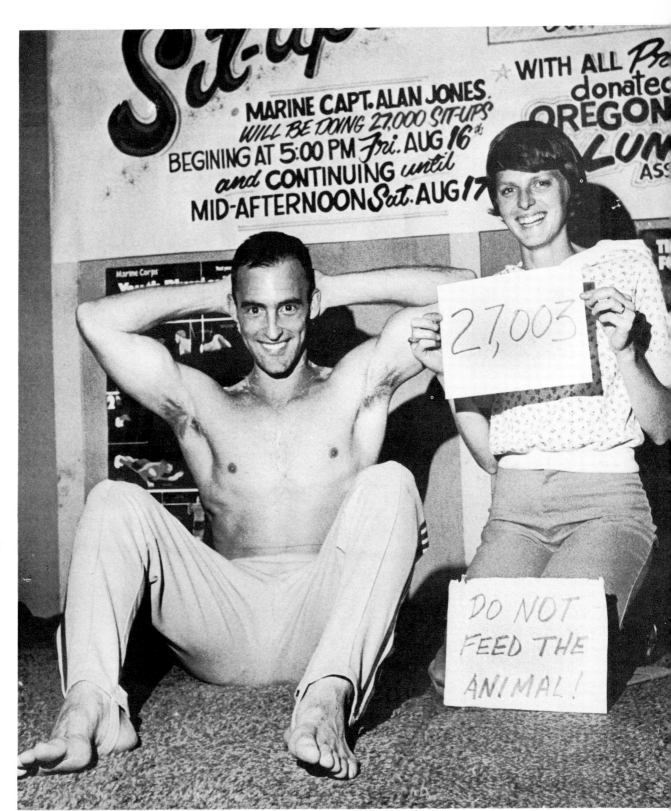

Marine Capt. Alan Jones did 27,003 sit-ups over a 24-hour period—yet his abs are barely noticeable.

The 15 Best

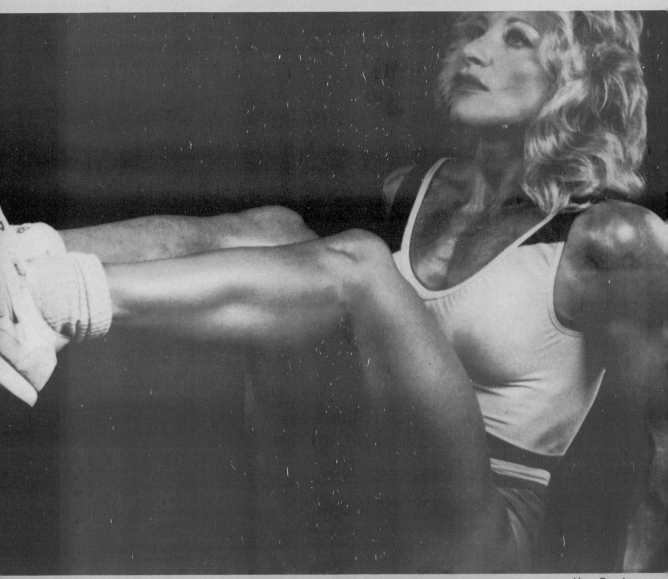

Kay Baxter

Abdominal Exercises

Every time you twist your body, raise your legs, or reach for something, the abdominal muscles are brought into play to some degree. They help us keep our balance and generally assist in most torso movements in one way or another. Over the years, I have experimented with literally hundreds of different abdominal exercises. The following exercises are, in my opinion, the most superior movements.

Dennis Tinerino has very symmetrical ab muscles.

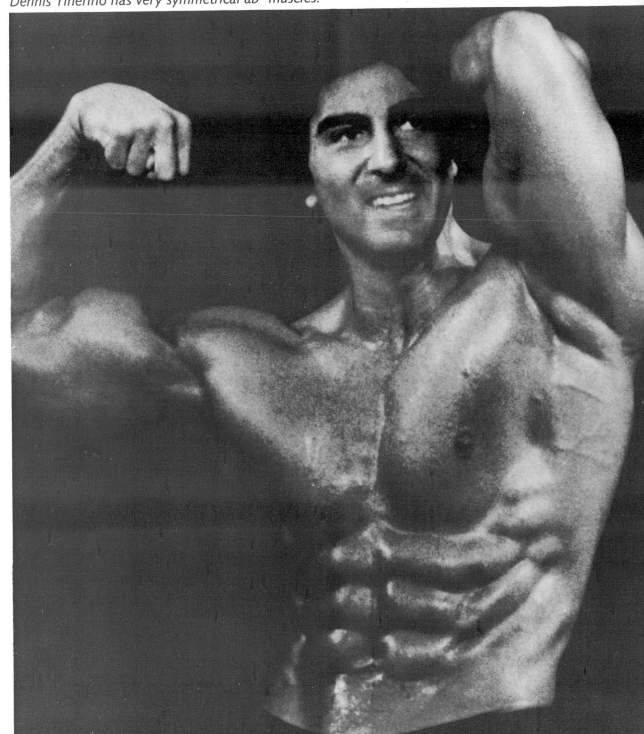

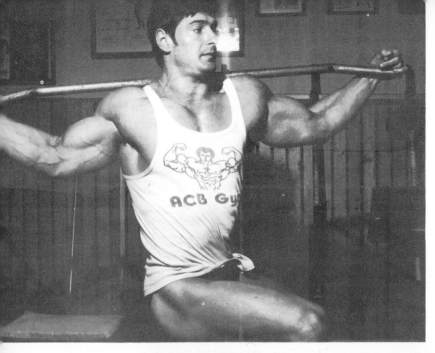

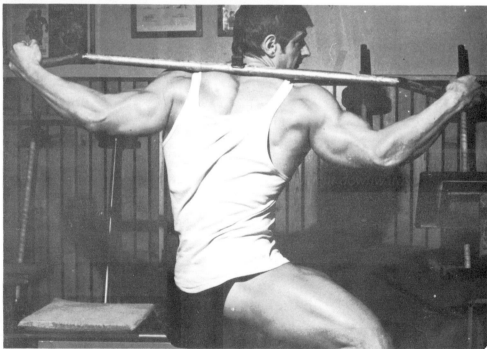

Petar Celik uses a bar from a lat machine to demonstrate seated twists.

Seated Twist (Side Abdominals/ Obliques)

Sit on a bench with a broomstick handle (or an empty barbell bar) across the back of your shoulders, held in place by your hands on either side. Start the exercise by twisting from side to side (moderate speed) concentrating on the side oblique muscles. Keep your head facing forward throughout the movement.

Hanging Leg Raise
(Lower Abdominals)

Grasp an overhead horizontal bar with your hands spread apart a little wider than your shoulders and hang straight downwards. Keeping your legs straight, raise both feet together as high as you can, then lower slowly (as opposed to dropping quickly) and repeat. You may also do this exercise by raising your bent knees as high as possible. Both ways work the abdominal wall vigorously.

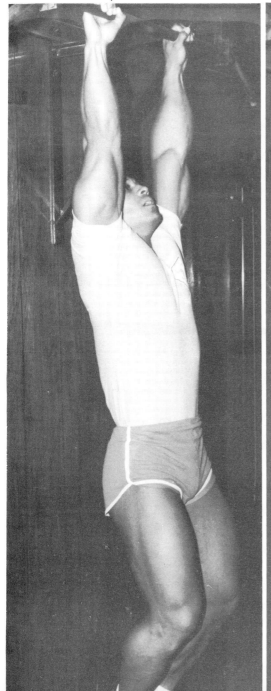

The beginning position of a hanging leg (or knee) raise by Mohamed Makkawy.

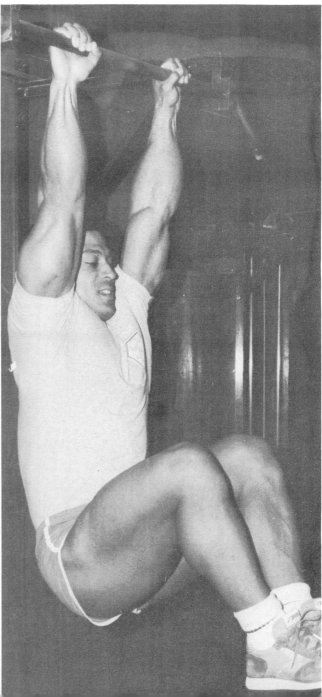

The completion of a hanging knee raise with bent knees.

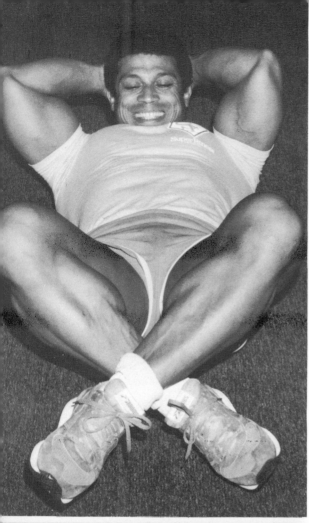

Crunch
(Middle Abdominals)

Lie on the floor on your back with your hands behind your neck. Raise your shoulders off the ground while at the same time raising your knees towards your head. Try to touch your elbows to your knees. Lower and repeat.

Mohamed Makkawy shows the beginning of the abdominal crunch . . .

. . . and the finish of the exercise.

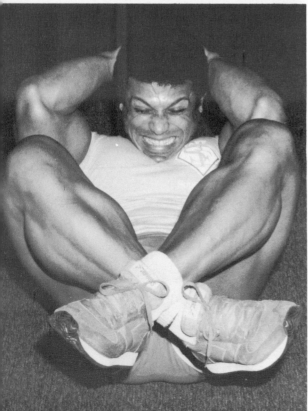

Roman Chair Sit-Up (Upper and Middle Abdominals)

Sit comfortably on a Roman chair apparatus. Lower rearwards until your body is parallel to the floor. Sit up and repeat. Some people prefer to use additional weight in this exercise. You can hold a weight disc on your chest during the exercise if you want to add resistance.

Carol Jurcovic extends her torso for a sit-up on a Roman chair.

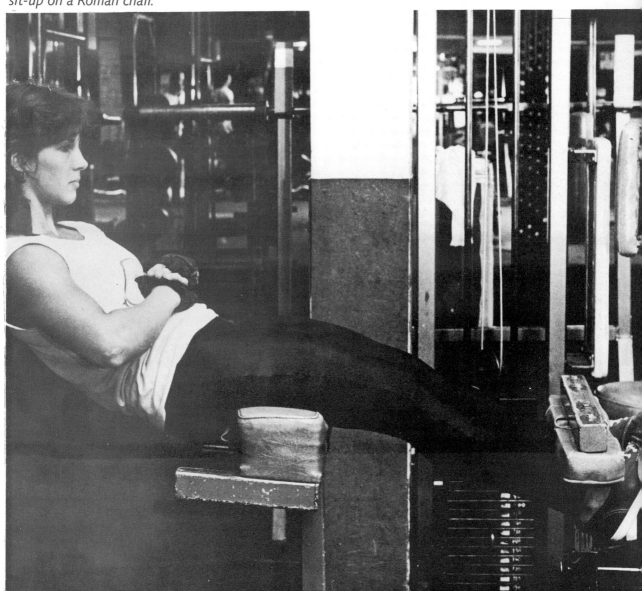

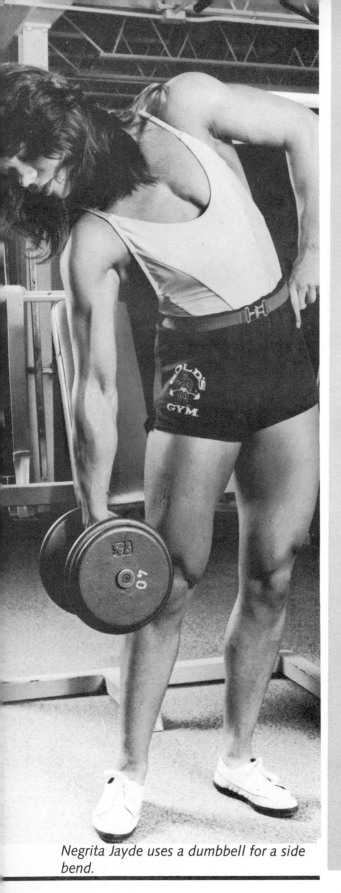

Negrita Jayde uses a dumbbell for a side bend.

Side Bend
(External Obliques)

Hold a dumbbell in one hand with your arm extended down the side of your body. Lean slightly rearwards and bend the torso from side to side, running the free hand (palm in) up and down the leg as you bend. (Do not do this exercise if you are naturally wide in the hips.) Change the dumbbell to the other hand and perform the same number of repetitions.

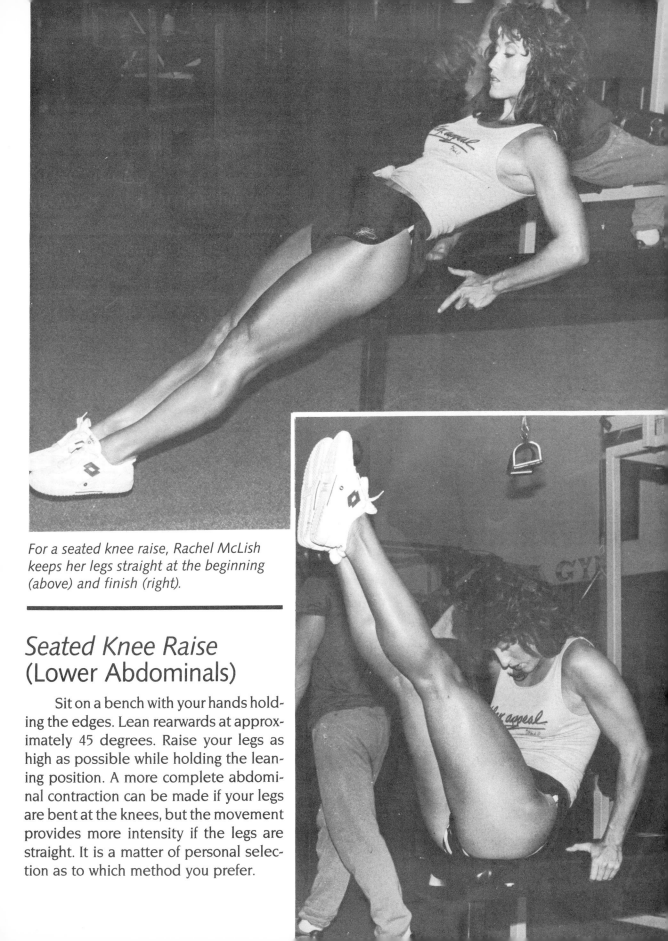

For a seated knee raise, Rachel McLish keeps her legs straight at the beginning (above) and finish (right).

Seated Knee Raise (Lower Abdominals)

Sit on a bench with your hands holding the edges. Lean rearwards at approximately 45 degrees. Raise your legs as high as possible while holding the leaning position. A more complete abdominal contraction can be made if your legs are bent at the knees, but the movement provides more intensity if the legs are straight. It is a matter of personal selection as to which method you prefer.

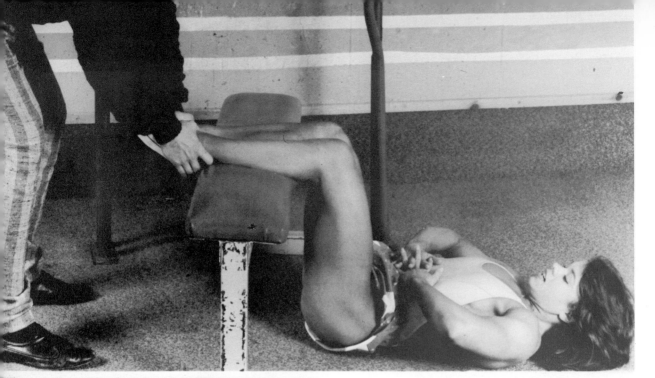

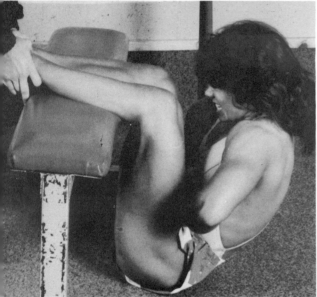

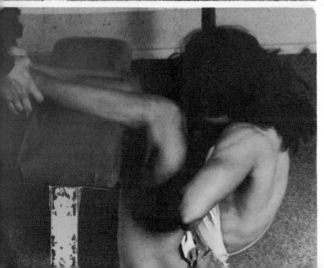

This three-photo sequence shows Negrita Jayde performing a bench crunch. Her hands could also be positioned behind her neck.

Bench Crunch (Upper and Middle Abdominals)

Lie on the floor and place your calves on top of a regular exercise bench in such a way that your thighs are perpendicular to the floor. Place your hands behind your neck (or on your stomach as illustrated) and raise your shoulders off the floor by vigorously contracting your abdominals. Lower and repeat. Another version of this movement is to keep your legs completely straight while crunching upwards. Bodybuilding champion Lynn Conkwright places her legs up against a wall (with her feet about 3 feet apart) for her unique performance of this movement.

Bent-Over Twist
(Side Abdominals/ Obliques)

You can perform this exercise either in the standing position or while seated. Bend over at the waist while holding a broomstick handle or an empty barbell bar. While maintaining the bent-forward position, proceed to twist from side to side. If you are not familiar with this exercise, you will not be able to twist much at first, but with practice you will develop plenty of flexibility.

Ms. Jayde illustrates a bent-over twist.

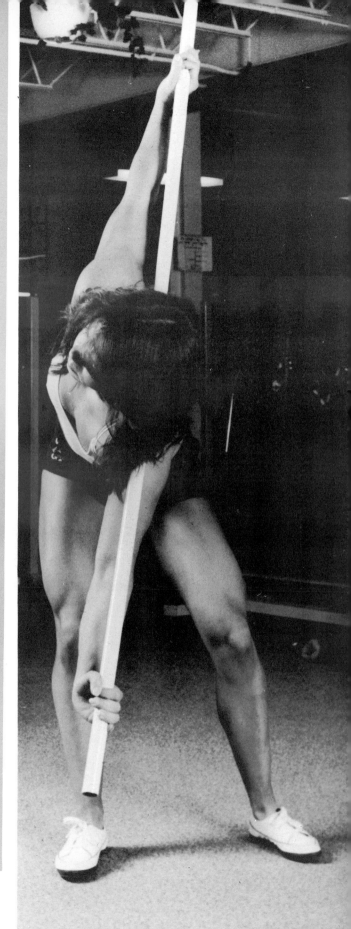

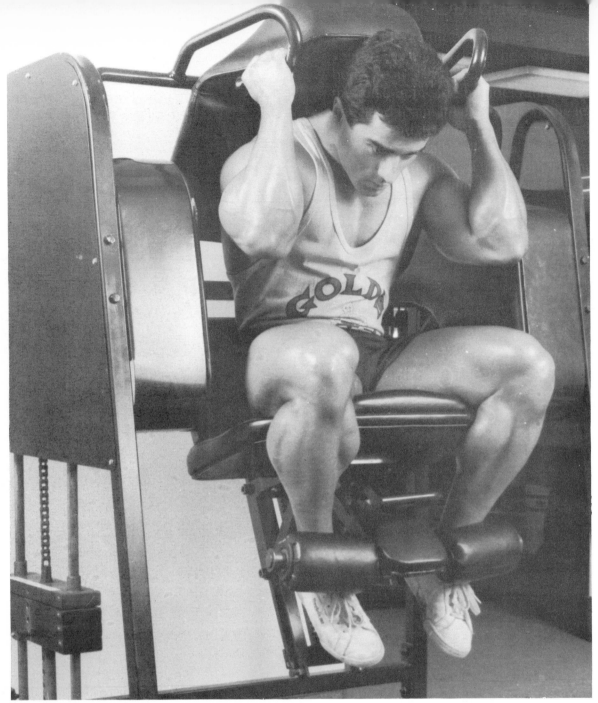

Steve Brisbois demonstrates a machine crunch.

Machine Crunch
(Middle Abdominals)

There are numerous machines which are specifically designed to give your midsection a workout. Most of these involve sitting in an upright position and then leaning forward, against a variable resistance from pads placed against your chest. You then return to the sitting position and repeat. Be sure not to use a too-heavy resistance until your body has gotten used to the action of an individual machine.

Knee Tuck
(Lower Abdominals)

Lie on your back with your hands (palms on the floor) under your buttocks. Raise your head off the floor. Lift both legs together, bending your knees as you raise them upwards. Bring your knees towards your face so that your hips raise slightly off the floor. Lower and repeat. This is a favorite exercise of former Ms. Olympia Rachel McLish.

Tom Platz does his version of a knee tuck, bringing his knees towards his chest.

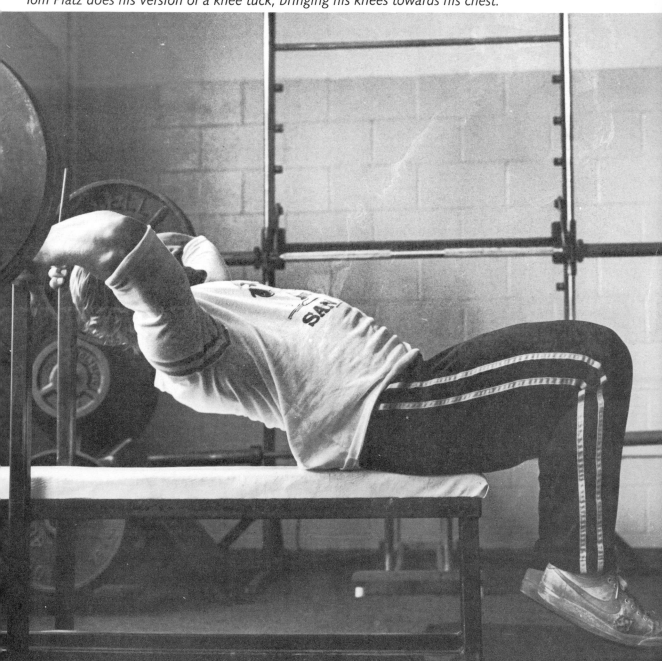

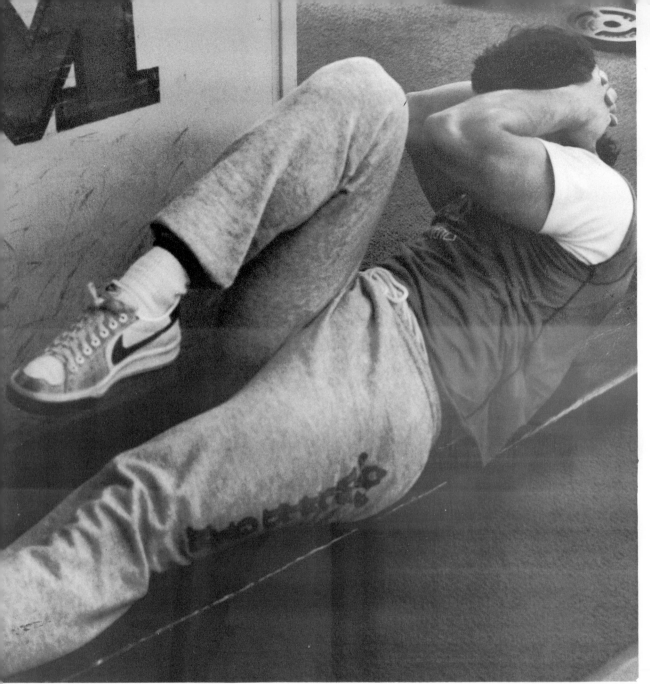

An alternate knee-raise crunch is done by Jon Jon Park.

Alternate Knee-Raise Crunch
(Entire Abdominals)

Lie on your back with your hands clasped behind your head, your feet together and toes pointed. Raise your right elbow and shoulder from the floor and at the same time lift your left knee (bending it fully as you lift it). Try to touch the knee with your elbow. Return to starting position. Next, lift the left elbow and shoulder while raising the right knee. Alternate for the desired number of repetitions.

Bent-Knee Partial Sit-Up (Upper and Middle Abdominals)

Lie on your back with your ankles crossed and thighs perpendicular to the floor. Clasp your hands behind your neck or hold them at the hip area. Raise your shoulders off the floor in a partial sit-up. Lower and repeat. Do not jerk your body upwards, but rather raise slowly by contracting your abdominals.

Gladys Portugues raises her torso slightly for a bent-knee partial sit-up in this two-photo sequence. She could also cross her ankles with her calves parallel to the floor.

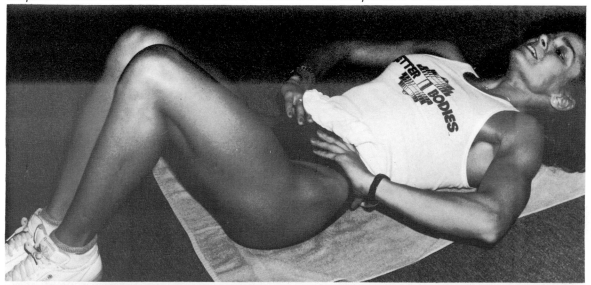

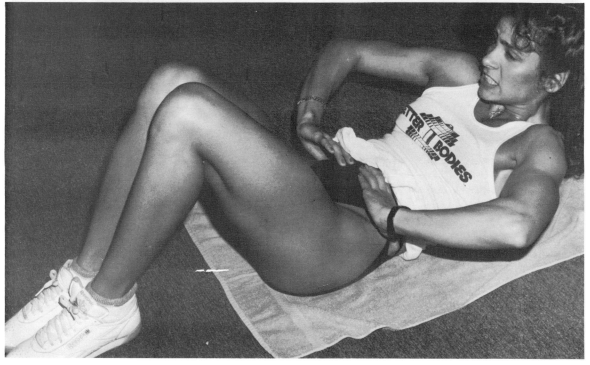

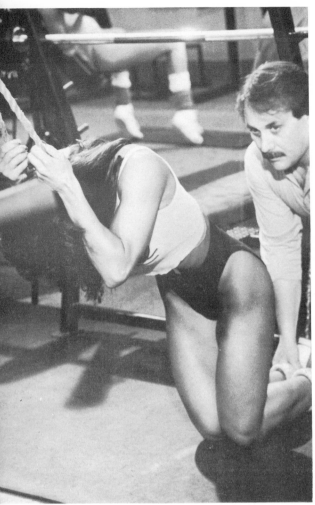

Rachel McLish holds a rope loop behind her head at the start of a cable crunch.

She concentrates on using her abdominals to pull the weight downwards.

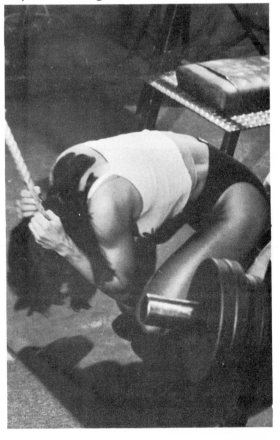

Cable Crunch (Middle Abdominals)

With your back towards a cable machine, hold an overhead cable behind your head with both hands while kneeling on the ground or on an exercise bench. Bend over forward while keeping the cable held tight in position. Raise up and repeat. You may require a training partner to hold your ankles down during the exercise.

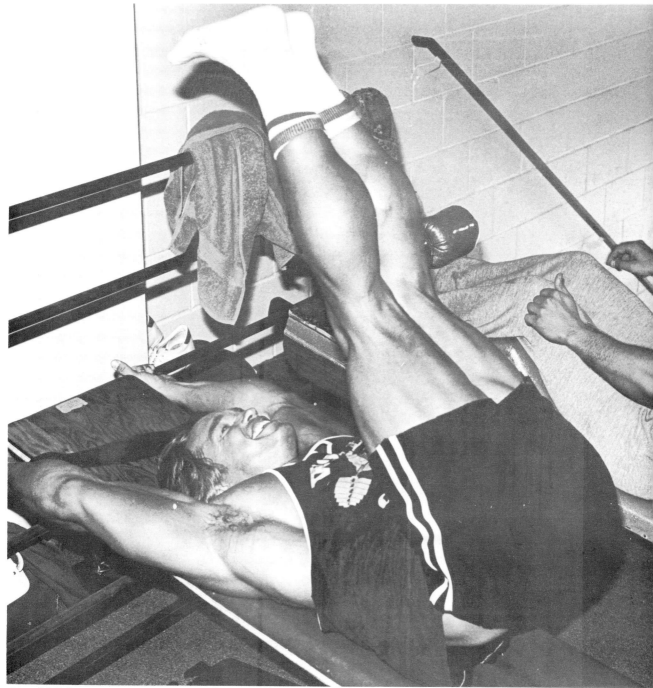

Arnold Schwarzenegger supports himself from above for an incline leg raise.

Incline Leg Raise
(Lower Abdominals)

Lie back on an incline bench at a 45-degree angle or less. Hold the bench with your hands near both sides of your head for support. Raise both legs together as far back as you can. It is optional whether you bend your knees or keep them straight. Lower and repeat.

Incline Bench Half Sit-Up
(Middle Abdominals)

Seat yourself on an incline bench that has an attachment to secure your feet in the upper position. A bent-leg position is superior to a straight-leg stance. Holding your hands behind your head, lift your shoulders off the bench. It is not necessary to sit all the way up, although some bodybuilders like doing so. Lower and repeat.

Charlie Thomas comes all the way up when he does sit-ups on an incline bench.

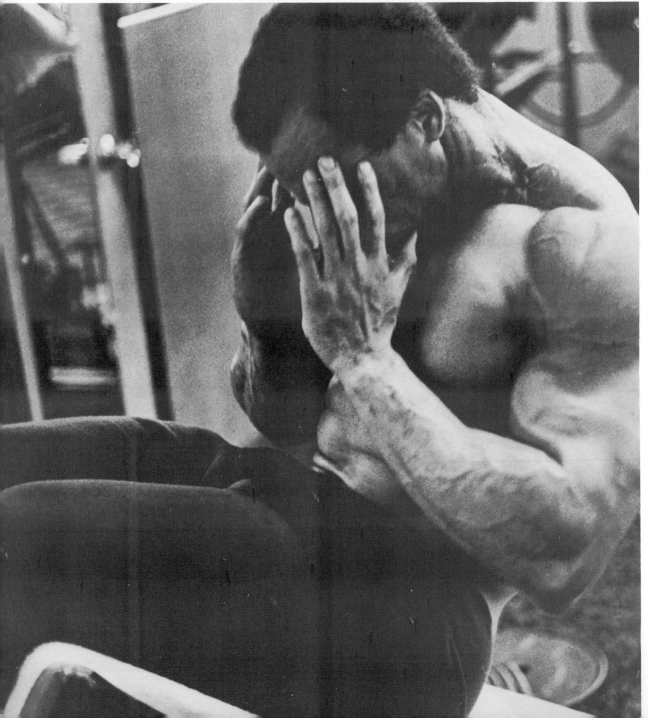

How Many Reps?

Just how many repetitions of an exercise should you do for your abs? It's a question with no single answer agreed to by all. Some people argue that it doesn't matter whether you do six or 60 reps, so long as the last few reps are difficult to complete. I do subscribe to this theory to an extent, but I still feel there are figures that can be offered for general advice.

The beginner or older person should usually keep to a system of 15–30 reps per set. For exercises such as broomstick twists or side bends without weight, the reps can be built up into the hundreds.

Bodybuilders who want to build a prize-winning physique should make a decision about what his or her particular needs are. Once you have decided which exercises you will be doing (to put emphasis on the upper, middle, or lower abdominals), you must decide whether you want to build bigger, more muscular abdominals or smaller, streamlined abdominals. If you already have large, chunky ab muscles, then I would suggest keeping to a program of relatively high reps using a variety of exercises. This will refine your midsection as you carve in that extra quality that results from working a muscle from different angles. Make all your reps over 20 per set.

In the case of the trainer who doesn't have abdominals that stand out in bold relief, I suggest that he or she perform repetitions between the 8–12 mark and that additional resistance is used in all exercises. When you add weight for waist exercises, make sure that you observe the following precautions:

1. Never use extra weight unless you have performed the exercise for several workouts without additional resistance.
2. Execute each exercise slowly and deliberately. Do not bounce or jerk during the performance. Strict style is imperative.
3. Make your weight increases gradual. It's better to add a pound or two of resistance each week than to add 20 pounds all at once.

How many reps do the champs do? It varies. Frank Zane regularly did 200 reps in his ab exercises. Zabo Kozewski, Bill Pearl, Candy Csencsits and Ed Guiliani worked by the clock, performing non-stop waist training for at least 25 minutes—up to 1,000 reps.

I remember watching Serge Nubret perform broomstick twists a month before competing (and winning) the NABBA Mr. Universe contest. He did the exercise for one hour non-stop. Tom Platz does literally hundreds of Roman chair sit-ups. He keeps going until his abs just can't do anymore. Carla Dunlap keeps her reps at around 50 per set (for three or four sets). Cory Everson is less structured in her program. As a contest approaches, she just progresses from one exercise to another, doing different amounts of reps until she has thoroughly worked her abs from numerous angles.

Several authorities (including Vince Gironda and Joe Weider) have pointed out that the abdominals require no more than 10–12 repetitions for maximum growth and tone, and that more repetitions are a waste of time. It is nevertheless true that the trial-and-error brigade of champion male and female bodybuilders have basically settled on performing between 15–30 reps for most of their ab exercises (see Abdominal Routines of the Champions).

Bodybuilding

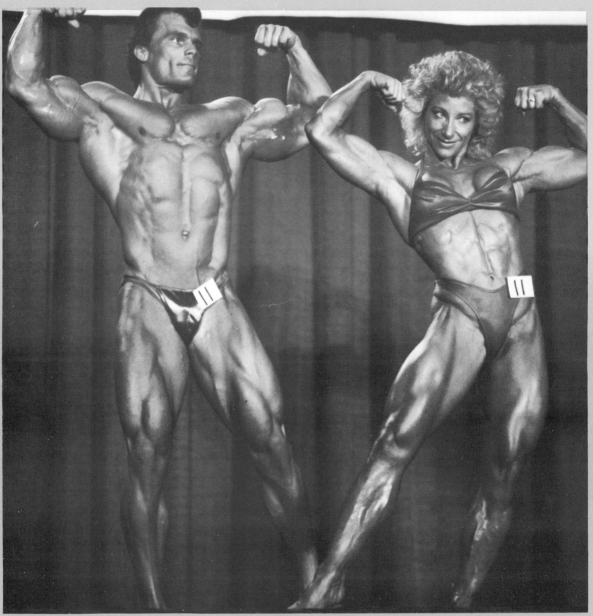

Gary Leonard and Kay Baxter

Beginners

W hen you start training, you have to remember to start slowly. If you use weights for an exercise, they have to be light weights. Where abdominal workouts are concerned, no weights at all should be used in the beginning. In fact, many advanced bodybuilders never use weights when performing waistline exercises.

Beginners to bodybuilding should never limit their workouts to just one body part. If you are new to progressive-resistance training, it is a much better idea to utilize an all-round routine that involves not only abdominal exercise but also trains the legs, shoulders, chest, arms, and back. The following is a suitable routine for beginners to bodybuilding.

Beginner's Routine

	Sets	Reps
Abdominals		
Crunch	1	× 12
Thighs		
Squat	1	× 15
Chest		
Bench Press	1	× 10
Shoulders		
Seated Press behind Neck	1	× 10
Back		
Bent-over Row	1	× 10
Calves		
Standing Calf Raise	1	× 15
Biceps		
Barbell Curl	1	× 10
Triceps		
Triceps Extension	1	× 12

As recommended, one set is quite enough to begin with. After a couple of

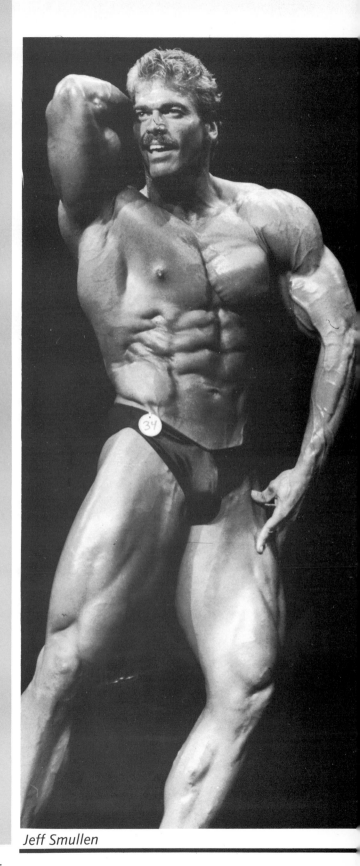

Jeff Smullen

weeks, as you improve in strength and condition, add more sets. Even more exercises can be introduced. The following is a guideline for those men and women who are beginning to train:

For the first two weeks, perform one set of your exercises only. After two weeks, perform two sets of each; after four to six weeks, do three sets. Obviously, due to the fact that everyone differs in age, condition, and tolerance for strenuous exercise, I cannot recommend precise sets, reps, and frequency figures. Be guided by how you feel. Re-

Rufus Howard holds a weight plate on his midsection to perform a Roman chair sit-up.

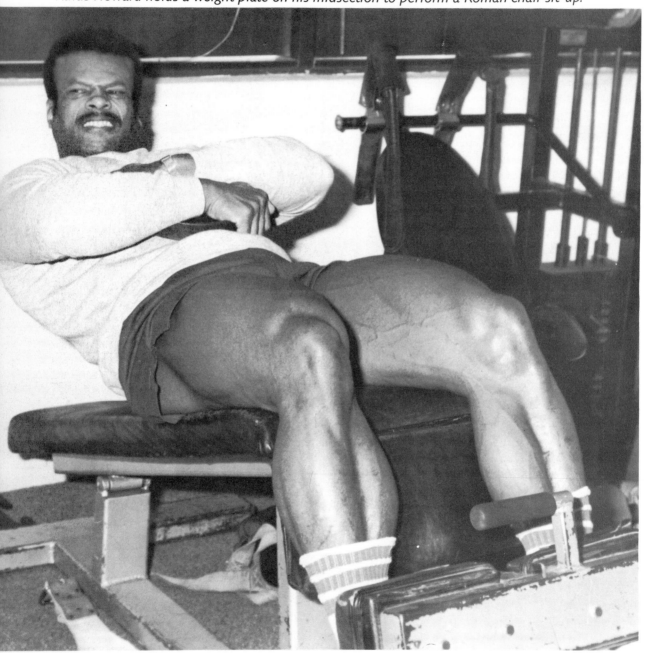

member above all that it is better to undertrain than to overtrain. If you suddenly throw an unconditioned body into excessive, vigorous abdominal exercise, you will not be able to get out of bed the next morning. Be prepared to progress slowly.

Vince Gironda points out in his book *Unleashing the Wild Physique* (Sterling Publishing Co., New York) that the abs can easily be overworked, throw an alarm if trained too hard, and will slow or shut down overall muscle gains. Gironda said: "Because they obtain the best blood supply in the body, the abdominals do not have to be worked with dozens of sets of high reps every day. This is most definitely not a good idea. You will smooth your abs out and subject your system to a degree of shock that can hinder gains if you overwork these sensitive muscles."

After you have passed through the beginner's stage of waist training, you will be able to perform two or three different exercises for three sets each. The following are two routines for the person with a very thin waist who wants to add all-round muscle thickness.

Abdominal Mass-Building Specialization

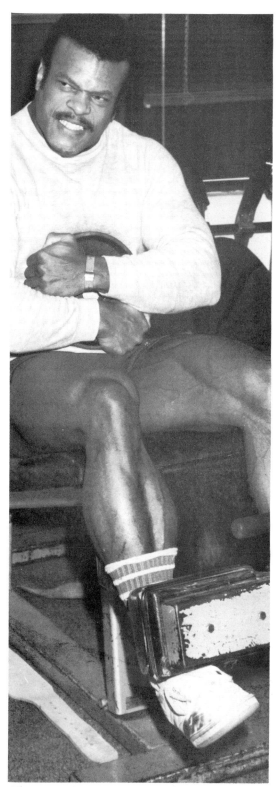

The completion of a Roman chair sit-up with additional weight.

Routine One	Sets	Reps
Side Bend (one dumbbell)	3	× 12
Roman Chair Sit-up (holding weight plate on chest)	3	× 12
Crunch (holding weight plate on chest)	3	× 10–12

Routine Two	Sets		Reps
Hanging Leg Raise	3	×	12
Bench Crunch (holding weight plate on chest)	3	×	12
Machine Crunch	3	×	12–15
Cable Crunch	2	×	12

As previously mentioned, add extra weight to an exercise only after you have performed that same exercise for several weeks without the use of additional weight. And when you do start adding weights, begin with the lowest poundage you can find. Build up the resistance over a period of weeks.

The following two routines should be considered for those who do not wish to add to the girth of their midsections. Note the repetitions are higher. There is more exercise variety and no additional weights are used.

Jon Jon Park does a crunch at the World Gym in Venice, California.

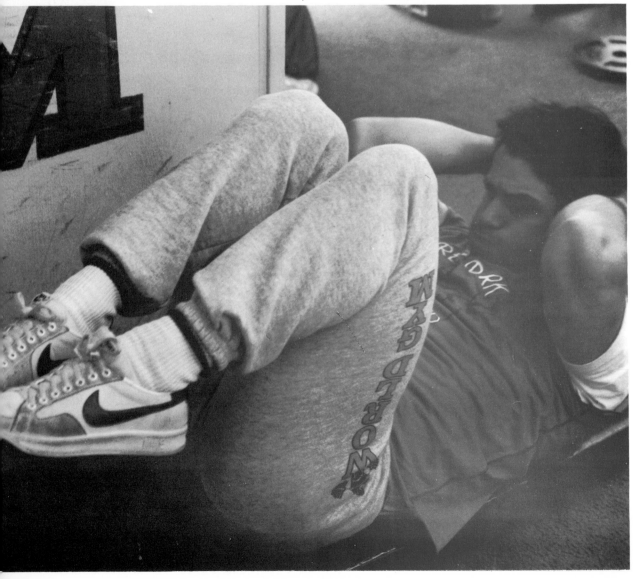

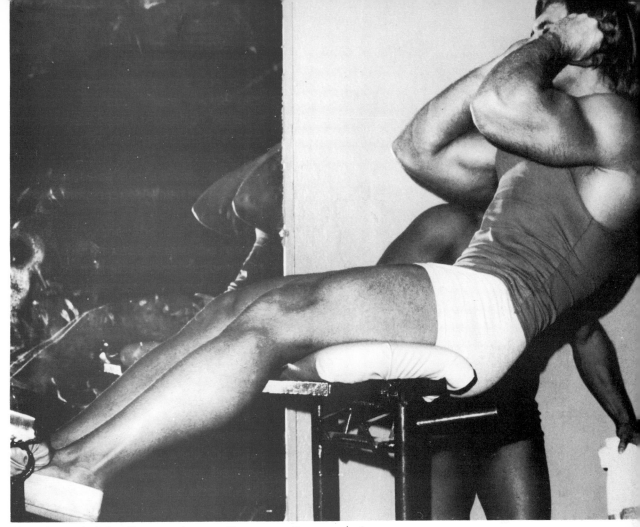

New Jersey's John Kemper does a sit-up on a Roman chair.

Abdominal Toning

Routine One	Sets	Reps
Hanging Leg Raise (with knees bent)	3	× 25
Crunch	3	× 20
Bent-over Twist	2	× 50
Seated Knee Raise	3	× 25

Routine Two	Sets	Reps
Twisting Roman Chair Sit-up	2	× 50
Side Bend (no weight)	2	× 100
Seated Twist	2	× 35
Knee Tuck	2	× 30

It is important that beginners understand from the very start that there are certain fundamental concepts about reducing fat around the midsection and building abdominals that show up in bold relief.

Remember that to be effective you must observe both the proper training regimen and a controlled diet. One will not work without the other. If you exercise hard, yet fail to follow a correct diet, then you will not achieve your goal of a slender, muscular midsection. Conversely, if you diet properly—taking care to reduce fats, starches, and overall calories—yet fail to exercise correctly, you will shed pounds, but you will not harden

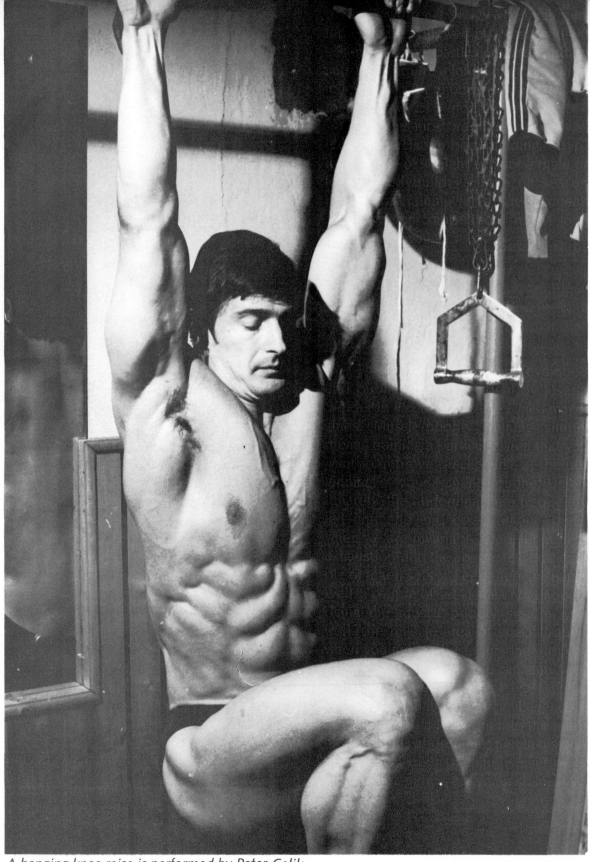

A hanging knee raise is performed by Peter Celik.

up or even tone your abdominal muscles. It is an absolute must, if you want the quickest and best possible results. It is the only way to win, yet literally millions of people who yearn to possess a trim, well-muscled waistline choose only one route.

By following the recommended exercise programs outlined in this book, you will build a rock-hard waistline and supportive abdominal muscles from your groin to the top of your sternum. Abdominal exercise in this case also has a secondary function—a calorie burner that helps to remove fat. However, this is not an effective way to burn off fat simply because most anaerobic exercises are poor calorie burners.

By adopting the suggestions in the nutrition chapter, your rows of abdominal muscles will start to show clearly. Eventually, they will stand out in bold relief.

A third aspect, which I will cover in detail in a later chapter, is the importance of a proper mental attitude. If you were satisfied with the way you look now, you wouldn't have purchased this book. On the other hand, you may be so far out of shape from overeating and laziness that right now you are carrying an enormous spare tire around your midsection. How did you get that way? Well, in all probability you developed a negative attitude towards your appearance and conditioning.

Accordingly, it's time to stop kidding yourself. There is no easy external solution. The answer is within you. The actual programs and diets are within these pages, but they are useless to you unless you nurture your resolve and dedication to attain success. Ultimately, it is your self-discipline that will give your midsection that winning look.

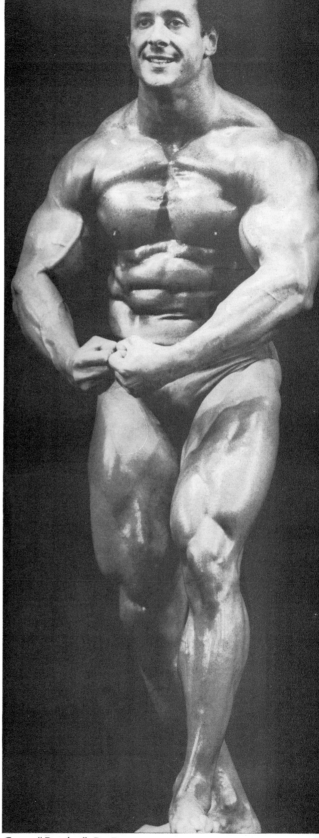

Greg "Rocky" DeFerro

Abdominal-
Training

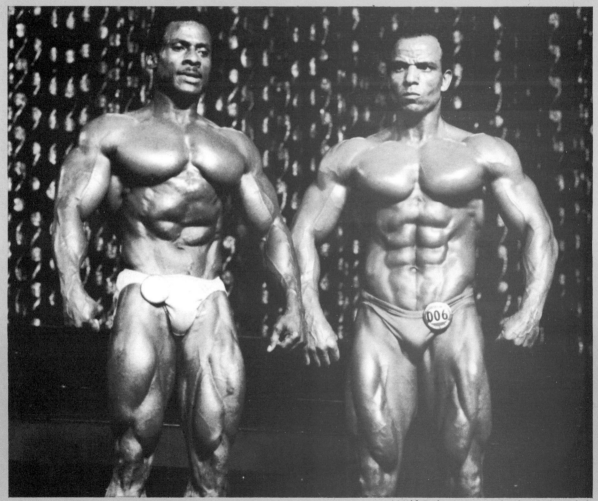

Wilf Sylvester and Ahmed Sadek

Principles

very muscle group has training techniques, systems, and principles that are more suited to it than others. For example, one training method that would not prove particularly beneficial to the abs is the rest-pause system, whereby one performs a single heavy repetition, rests for twenty seconds, then performs a second, a third, etc., each after a brief pause. The heavyweight single reps involved in rest-pause training are not suited to the waistline area.

Basically, the abs are a high-rep muscle, which translates into the recommendation that you never perform less than ten reps per set. Many experienced bodybuilders like to perform many reps for their abs. Men like Frank Zane, Zabo Kozewski, Ed Guiliani, Bill Pearl, and Tom Platz have experimented with rep numbers going into the hundreds. And their results have been most fruitful.

The abdominal area can be injured if it is subjected to too much overload, especially if this is done when the muscles are not fully warmed up. Because injury is no stranger to the abdomen, I would never suggest that you use forced reps or negative reps, both of which are principles utilized only when you cannot complete another repetition with your own muscle power. The following are some methods you can use to benefit the abdominal region.

Straight Sets

Let's say you perform a dozen abdominal crunches without stopping. As you should already know, each count is known as a repetition. Each time you finish a certain number of repetitions—whether it be ten, twenty, or two hun-

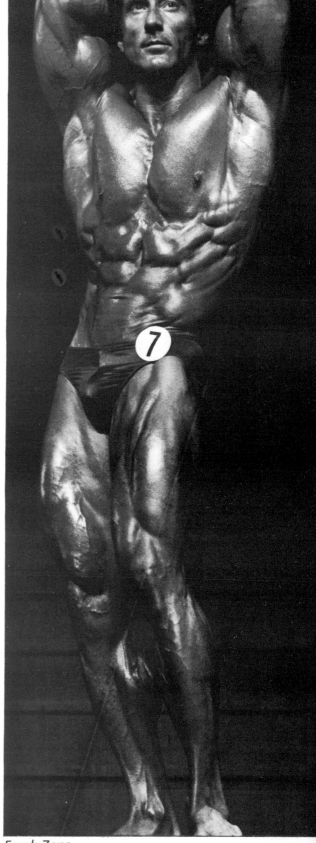

Frank Zane

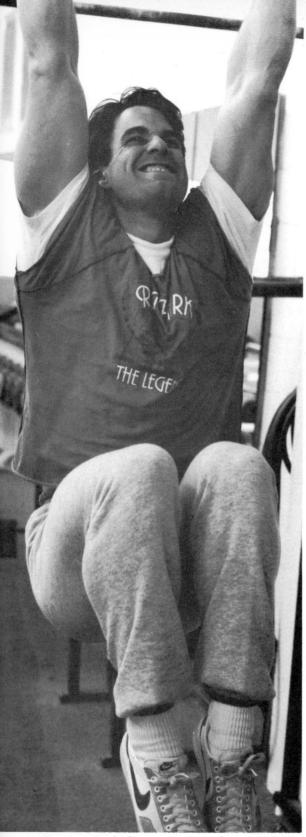
Jon Jon Park demonstrates a hanging knee raise.

dred—that group of non-stop reps is known as a set. Three sets of twelve repetitions is written 3 × 12. When you perform one set, followed by a rest of 30–90 seconds (some particularly demanding sets may require a longer rest) and then follow that with another set, and so on, this is known as performing *straight sets*.

It is the most frequently used system of exercise in bodybuilding. A typical routine of straight sets for a male or female bodybuilder in the off season (when not training for a specific peak condition for competition) might look like the following:

	Sets		Reps
Hanging Leg Raise	4	×	15
Crunch	3	×	20
Side Twist	2	×	50

Muscle Priority

This principle has been developed and publicized a great deal by Joseph Weider in *Flex* and *Muscle & Fitness* magazines. Muscle-priority training simply means training a particular area that you want to improve quickly first, at the beginning of your training routine. Unfortunately, the abdominals are frequently left until the end of a workout. That's when we are invariably tired, if not near exhaustion, and the abs are tossed a couple of token sets to keep them in shape. Well, a couple of sets is just not enough. Using the muscle-priority system, you work the muscle area of specialization when you are freshest, bursting with enthusiasm and energy. You can start your ab workout, performing at least 15–20 minutes of quality training. Legendary bodybuilder Bill Pearl got into the habit of training his abdominals first in his routine. He has been training over 40 years and his waistline is always in shape.

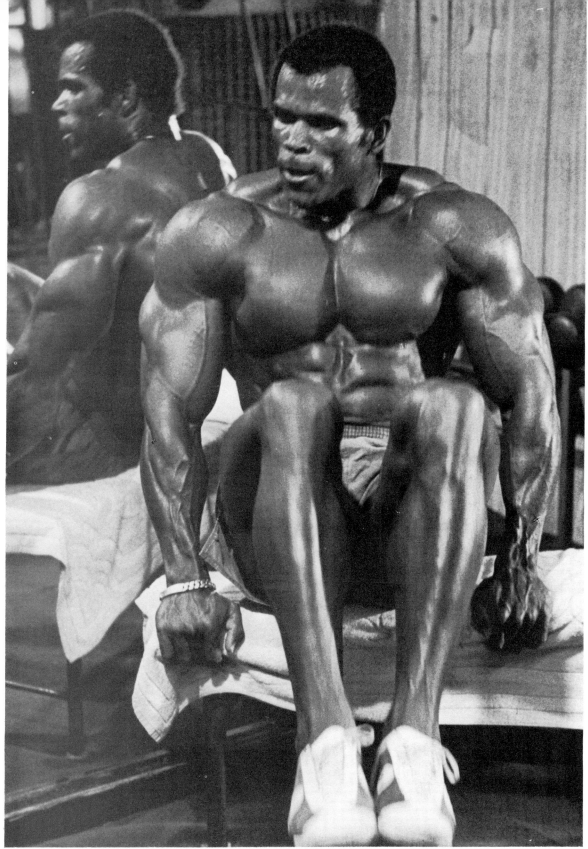

Serge Nubret does a seated knee raise.

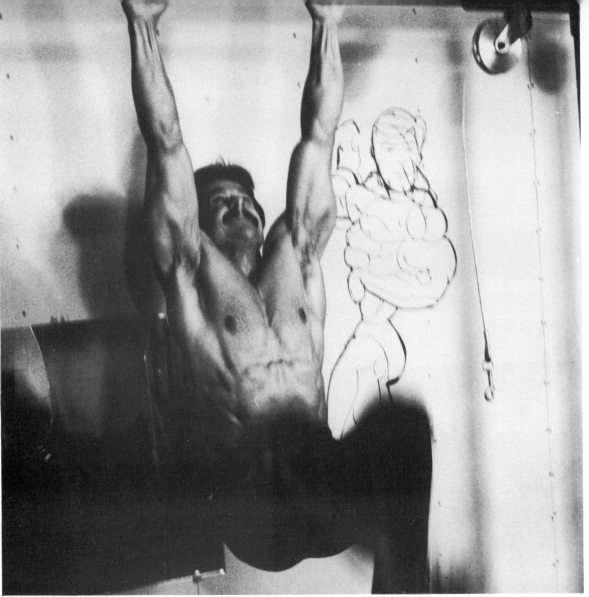

Anibal Lopez of New York City goes to work on his abs.

Isotension

As the name implies, isotension involves the tensing and flexing of the muscles while exercising. The principle can also be applied at times when you are not exercising, while at your office desk, in school, or in front of your bathroom mirror. Merely flexing your abdominals can build and tone them. One word of warning: When using this method, start moderately and build up both the effort you put into flexing your abs and the duration of each flex. Too much too soon may cause the muscles to cramp up—definitely not something you want to happen while driving in traffic.

Peak Contraction

This condition is only achieved in certain exercises in which the best (or hardest) contraction coincides with the end of the exercise movement. For example, let's examine the sit-up exercise performed with gravity boots. You begin the exercise by hanging upside down (using special boots attached to a horizontal bar). As you sit up from this upside-down position, the greatest effort (peak contraction) comes as you complete the sit-up. Peak-contraction movements come with that little bit extra, and consequently have the potential to make you work a little bit more. Some trainers like to hold the peak-contraction position for a two-second count. This, of course, increases the intensity of each repetition.

Actually, quite a few abdominal exercises are peak-contraction movements. Movements like regular sit-ups, Roman chair sit-ups, and leg raises are not peak-contraction exercises, but crunches, bench crunches, and dumbbell side bends are.

Giant Sets

Giant sets are sometimes known as compound sets, and they work well for the abdominal muscles. It is an advanced form of exercising because the muscles are worked continuously from different angles. The bonus is that when you perform giant sets, you save considerable time.

A giant set is the consecutive performance of four (or even five) exercises for one body part. You only rest after you have performed one set of each exercise. Then you perform the complete cycle again. For example an entire abdominal routine might be the following (which should be performed three times).

Abdominal Giant Set	Reps
Hanging Leg Raise	20
Crunch	15
Knee Tuck	25
Roman Chair Sit-up	50

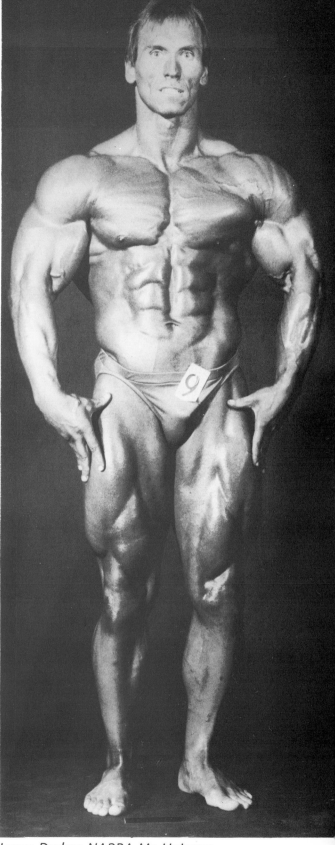

Lance Dreher, NABBA Mr. Universe

47

Abdominal-Specialization Routines

John Terilli

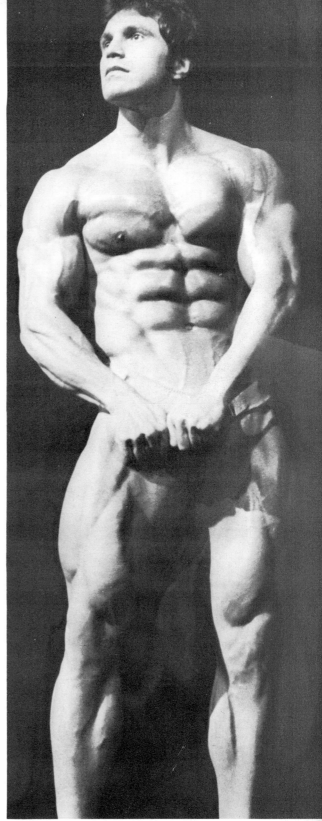

uilding your body is a multi-faceted task. Like a sculptor, we are artists with the ability to shape our bodies. Of course, we are limited by our genetics, natural shape, bone structure, and allocation of muscle cells, but the sculptor is also limited by the grain in his wood, the softness and texture of his stone, and the size and shape of his working material.

The bodybuilder's tools are not the mallet and chisel, but the exercise routines and diet plans we have at our disposal. It is the way we use these tools that determines whether we create a poor body, a so-so image, or an outstanding work of art. Look at building your body like a diamond cutter who starts with a rough stone and with very skillful use of cutting and shaping techniques, he brings out a priceless sparkling jewel. The process has to be attacked from different angles to make the ultimate impact. The right cuts must be made.

It is important to train your abdominals from different angles, too, and vital that correct diet be used. You will never regret taking the time to think about how to work your midsection to bring about the best results.

Let's clarify a fact about abdominal muscles right here. You cannot change the shape of your abdominal wall. Some people have even rows of muscles in their midsections, while others have scattered, uneven layers of abdominal development. Judges may prefer to see even rows of abdominal development, but generally speaking, there is not much advantage in having your abs laid out in straight rows. They look neater, of course, when they are straight, but a judge will vote for the sharpest and most defined abs rather than ones that are straight.

Straight abs are the hallmark of Joe Nazario.

The easiest part of the abdominals to develop is the upper area since most exercises affect this part more than any other. The most difficult area to bring out is the lower reaches, below and around the navel. Only a few select exercises work this part.

James Mathé of France was an early bodybuilder who concentrated on abdominal development.

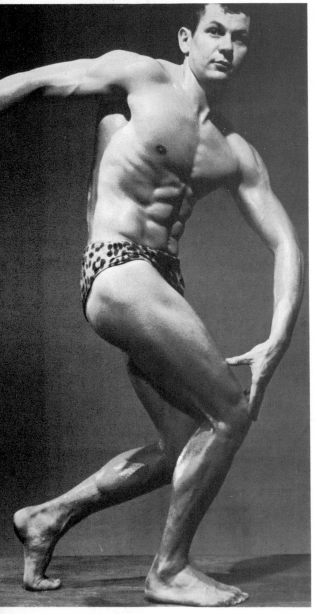

For as long as I can remember, and this holds true for today, the best abdominal development seems to come from French bodybuilders. They follow their own traditions. It's the same with their bodybuilding. On the numerous occasions when I have trained in France, I have never seen anyone working out with heavy squats. They still believe heavy squats are bad for the heart, and they don't try to develop massive type thighs. All French physique stars have underdeveloped legs by American, German, and British standards. In regard to abdominal training, the French way of thinking is advanced over the rest of the world. French bodybuilders believe that it's very important to develop their abdominals evenly. They consciously strive to build the upper, middle, and lower areas to the same degree. This extra attention pays off. Accordingly, the best abdominals today belong to Gerard Buinoud, Serge Nubret, Jacques Neuville, all of France.

Of course, there are some magnificent sets of abdominals outside the French community. For instance, people like Mohamed Makkawy, Inger Zetterqvist, Corinna Everson, Tony Pearson, John Hnatyschak, Eduardo Kawak, Dinah Anderson, and Bev Francis all have wonderful abdominal development, but the touch of class invariably has that French connection. In fact, during the fifties and sixties, the French bodybuilders believed the midsection to be the *most* important body part, while the Americans considered it to be the *least* important. The American bodybuilders were developing huge thighs, pecs, and arms, while the French were going for abs, shoulders, and lats. Today things are evening up more, but the French still

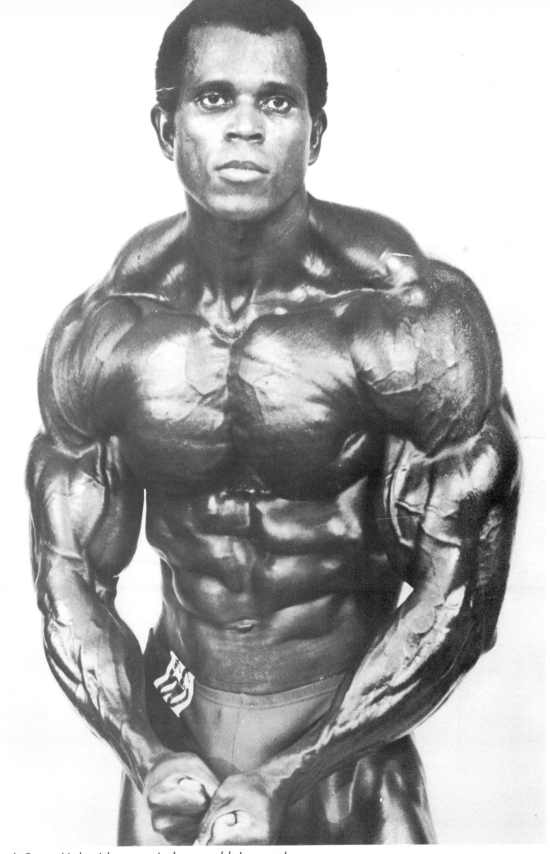

France's Serge Nubret has great abs—and lots more!

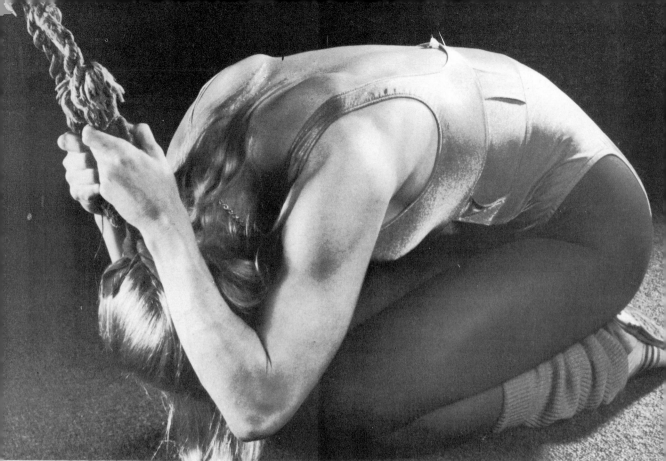

Shelley Gruwell performs a cable crunch.

have the edge when it comes to midsection perfection.

Make up your mind now to have the most evenly built, deeply ridged abdominal muscles possible. Balance up your midsection so that the lower areas are equally developed to the middle, side, and upper areas. In this way, whether you are seen on the beach or under the lights at a bodybuilding contest, you will be secure in the knowledge that your abdominals are as perfectly built as is humanly possible.

Upper Abdominals

The upper area of the abdominal wall starts just below the low line of the pectoral (chest) muscles. Frequently, this area is developed more than the middle and lower areas. I have only seen the upper area superseded by middle and lower abdominals a few times in my life. The following routines concentrate the action into the upper abdominals.

Upper Abdominal Specialization

Routine One	Sets	Reps
Roman Chair Sit-up (only going halfway down)	3	× 15–20
Bench Crunch	3	× 15
Cable Crunch	3	× 15

Routine Two	Sets	Reps
Bent-knee Partial Sit-up	3	× 15–20
Alternate Knee-raise Crunch	3	× 15–20
Bench Crunch	3	× 15–20

Middle Abdominals

Developing the middle abdominal region requires specific exercises, but there is always some overspill effect. In other words, when you work the middle abs, there will be some benefit to both the upper and the lower sections. The following routines put the main emphasis of exercise on the middle abdominal region.

Middle Abdominal Specialization

Routine One	Sets	Reps
Roman Chair Sit-up (full movement)	2	× 50
Crunch	3	× 15
Bench Crunch	3	× 25

Routine Two	Sets	Reps
Machine Crunch	3	× 15–20
Bent-knee Partial Sit-up	3	× 12
Incline Bench Half Sit-up	3	× 12

Andrea LaMantia shows how she does a sit-up on a Roman chair.

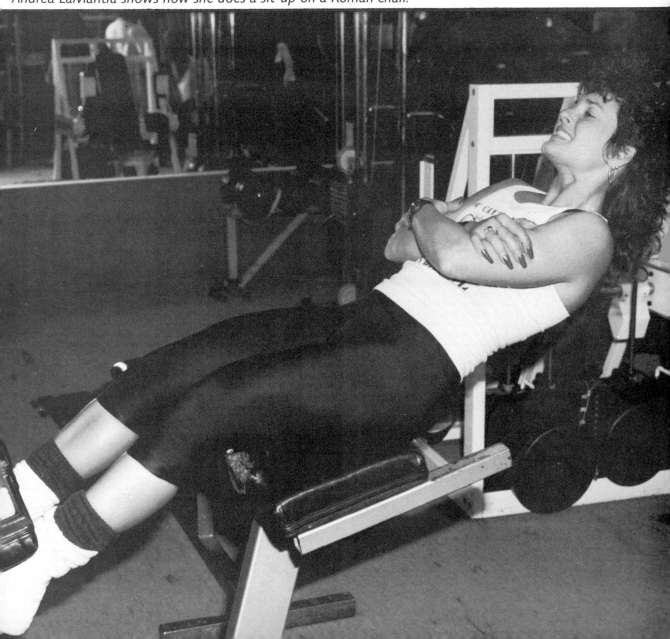

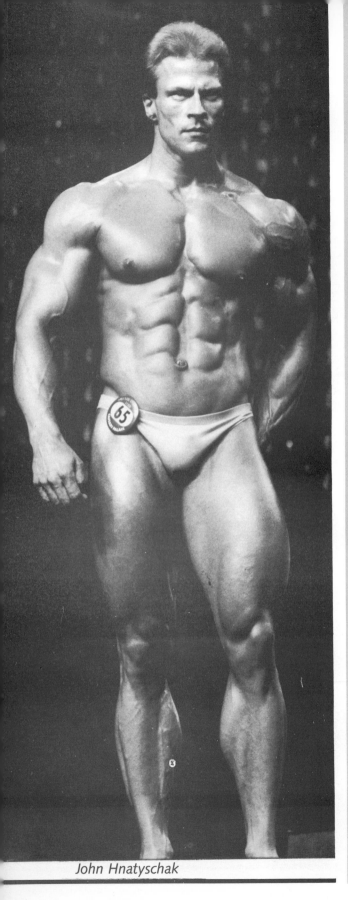
John Hnatyschak

Lower Abdominals

This is the bugaboo of most body-builders. Everyone has two or three rows of ab muscles above the navel (most have three). However, it is the single layer *below* the navel that is traditionally the hardest to develop. Some star body-builders are completely lacking in this section. Look at the various pictures in the magazines and you will see for yourself. There is a flatness with hardly a dimple of muscle. When you see these body-builders on stage at a show, you get the feeling that there should be something else there. Many are not even aware of it, yet they are stymied when they are beaten by another bodybuilder who has taken the trouble to build lower abs. The following routines concentrate on building the lower part of your frontal midsection.

Lower Abdominal Specialization

Routine One	Sets		Reps
Hanging Leg Raise (slowly with no swinging)	3	×	15
Roman Chair Sit-up (stretch all the way back)	3	×	25
Knee Tuck	3	×	25

Routine Two	Sets		Reps
Seated Knee Raise	3	×	15–20
Incline Leg Raise	3	×	15–20
Alternate Knee-raise Crunch	3	×	15–20

Side Midsection

The sides of the waist often accumulate fat, especially as we get older. The obliques lose their tone and the spare tire around the waist robs us of that tight-

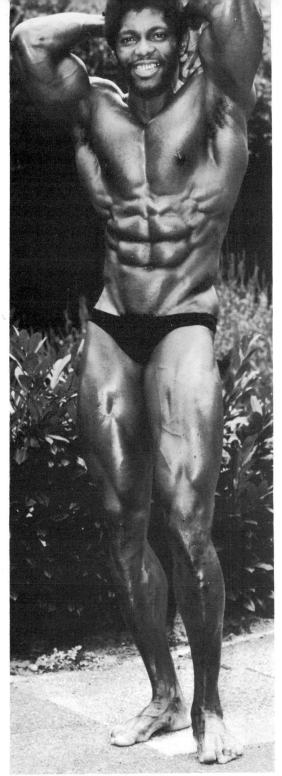

Serge Lerus

moved by taking in fewer calories. The exercise part is the toner and conditioner. The following specialized routines work the sides of the waistline.

Side Midsection Specialization

Routine One	Sets	Reps
Twisting Roman Chair Sit-up	3	× 15
Side Bend (each side)	3	× 20–25

Routine Two	Sets	Reps
Bent-over Twist	2	× 50–100
Alternate Knee-raise Crunch	2	× 20
Seated Twist	2	× 50–100

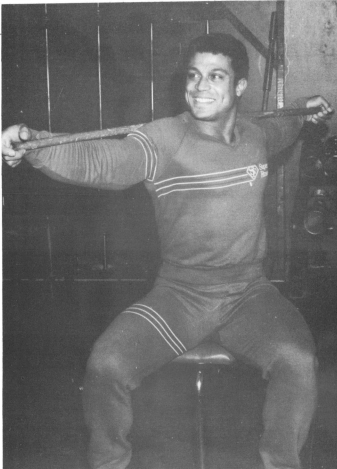

Mohamed Makkawy does seated twists.

tapered look. It makes our shoulders and back appear narrower. As for the other parts of the abdomen, fat is best re-

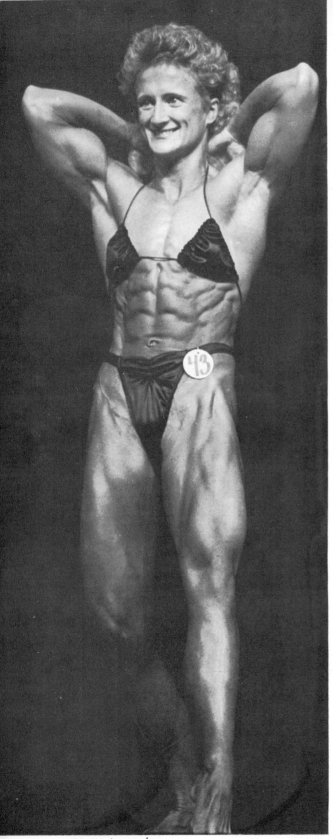

Mary Jerumbo

Women's Abdominal Training

Some women who feel they work their abs as hard as they possibly can still are disappointed with the results of their labors. They long to have the well-defined abdominals that many top male bodybuilders possess. What can they do?

The answer may lie partially in the fact that women's body fat percentages are somewhat higher than men's. It could be argued that it is not "normal" for a woman's abdominals to show. Well, the truth is that many women possess ab muscles that show deep, clear ridges— and some of these women don't even train to get them. However, they do have low body fat levels. If your abs show, then you can be pretty sure there's not too much fat under your skin, at least around your midsection area. Women who desire well-defined abs must train them hard and double up on their efforts to keep their body fat levels at a lower percentage than usual. This requires calorie control. (See the chapter on Diets for a Fat-free Waistline.)

There's no need for women to use heavy weights when training their midsections. Use higher reps with little or no extra resistance. Make sure that when you perform exercises involving twists and turns, do the movement with a minimal amount of momentum. Focus on the area of the abs that a particular exercise is designed to work. For example, if you perform bent-knee leg raises for your lower abs, then concentrate on making your lower abs *feel* the movement as you do the exercise. The same goes for those twists. Make the external obliques drag your torso around each repetition. This

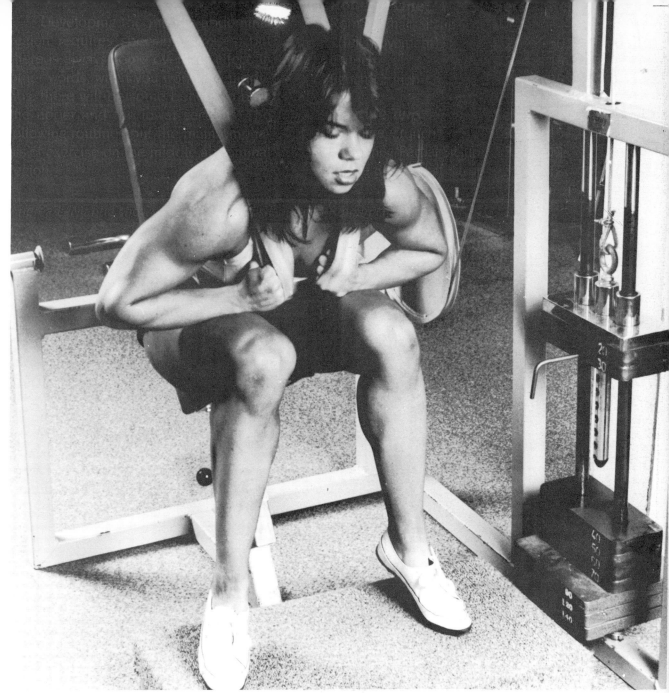

Machine crunches as performed by Canada's Negrita Jayde.

not only builds more size and tone, but also uses up more calories. The net result is a sharper-looking midsection.

If you have positively decided that your abdominal region is absolutely your worst and most out-of-shape body part, then you may want to take sterner measures and perform your midsection exer-

cises first in your routine, while you are full of energy. The abdominal region is one muscle group in which you cannot easily use too much variety. It would therefore be quite in order to select five, six, seven, or more different ab exercises, and to perform one set of each, with minimum rest between sets, all at the begin-

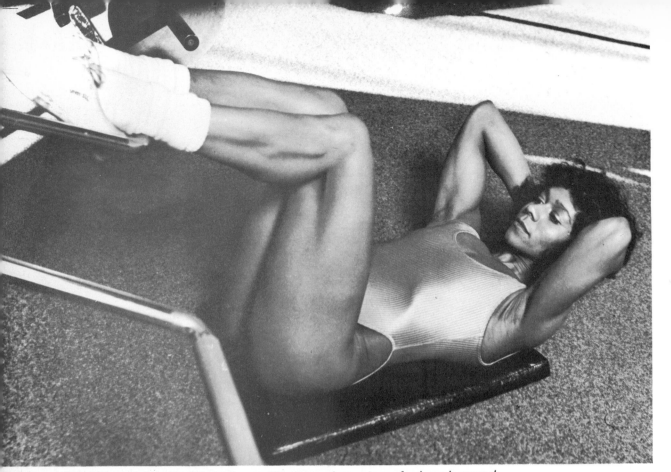

This two-photo sequence shows Kim Fonza's version of a bench crunch.

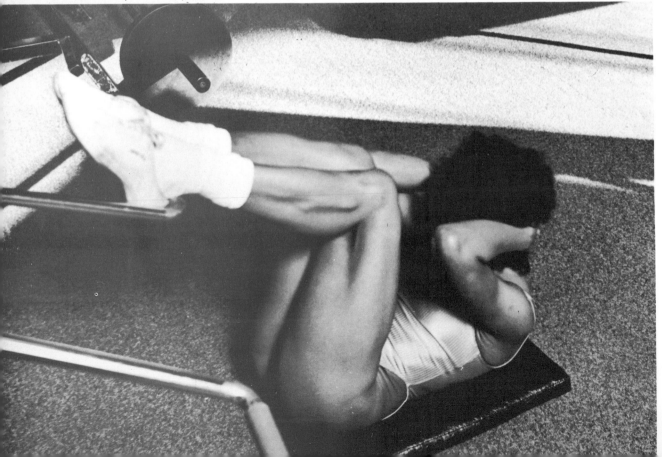

ning of your workout. This will stimulate your abs to the limit because time is on your side, as opposed to working them at the end of a workout when you may be running out of time and energy. Finally, training the abs first in your routine is a wonderful way of warming up the entire body.

The following abdominal routines for beginning female bodybuilders should be performed for one set of each exercise with no rest between sets. For intermediates, perform three giant sets of each complete with no rest between exercises but a brief rest between giant sets. For advanced female trainers, perform four giant sets of the complete routine.

Women's Beginning Ab Routine

	Sets	Reps
Roman Chair Sit-up	1	× 15–25
Hanging Knee Raise	1	× 15
Bench Crunch	1	× 15–20
Side Twist (with bar across shoulders)	1	× 200

Women's Intermediate Ab Routine

	Giant Sets	Reps
Knee Tuck	3	× 25
Crunch	3	× 15–20
Bent-over Twist	3	× 30

Women's Advanced Ab Routine

	Giant Sets	Reps
Twisting Roman Chair Sit-up	4	× 10–15 minutes
Seated Knee Tuck	4	× 10 minutes

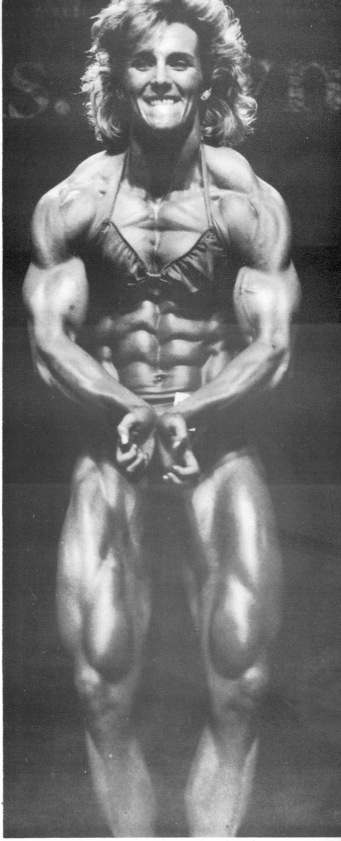

Bev Francis has the most muscular abs of any woman.

Winning

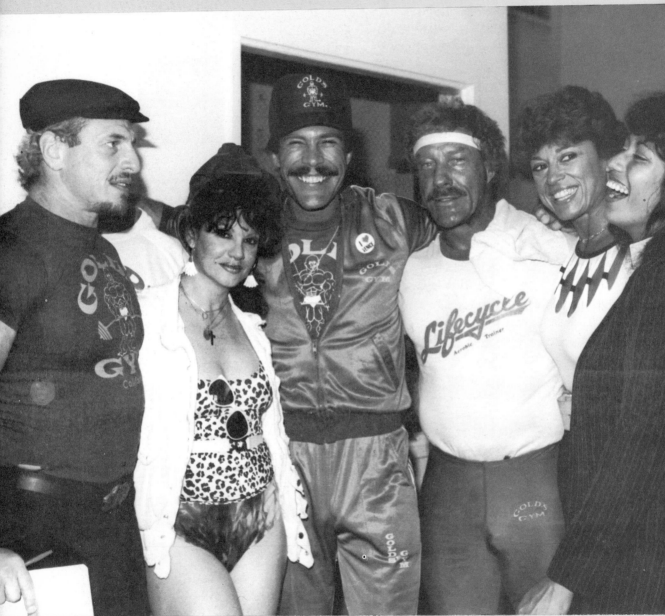

Don Ross, Lisa Lyon, Pete Grymkowski, Kent Kuehn, Fran Jeffries, and Linda Reyes.

Mental Attitude

Simply wishing for a better body is not enough. Former Mr. Olympia Franco Columbu said that the strongest and most important muscle is between our ears. Your mind dictates your achievements. If you can see yourself as a success, then you can mentally program yourself to reach the highest levels. Only your mind can harness your progress. Your attitude in relation to building super abdominals is important because you have to follow a two-point plan: 1. You must train the midsection regularly, even when it seems rather boring. 2. You have to keep a constant eye on your calorie consumption. A couple of weeks of eating too heartily can rob your midsection of that ultra-ripped sharpness.

If you are bored or undermotivated, you will have to consciously fire up your mind, to create an artificial enthusiasm until results become evident. When results show themselves in a positive way, you will find that your enthusiasm for training will increase naturally. Nothing makes us want to train harder than the experience of seeing tangible gains. On the other hand, a passive attitude about training, the lack of a forceful drive for achievement, can leave you in the middle of the gym with nowhere to go. If you do not have that hunger for improvement, you will never make much progress.

Other individuals may be plagued by overenthusiasm. This, too, can be an awesome burden. Overenthusiasm can lead to disappointment and frustration because results come too slowly. You may train too hard for too long and throw yourself into a sticking point. Muscles can only take so much shock treatment, and the abdominals are more sensitive to the

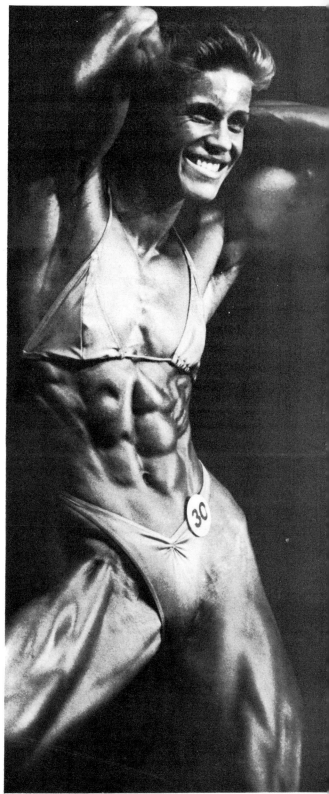

Anja Langer of Germany has amazing abs.

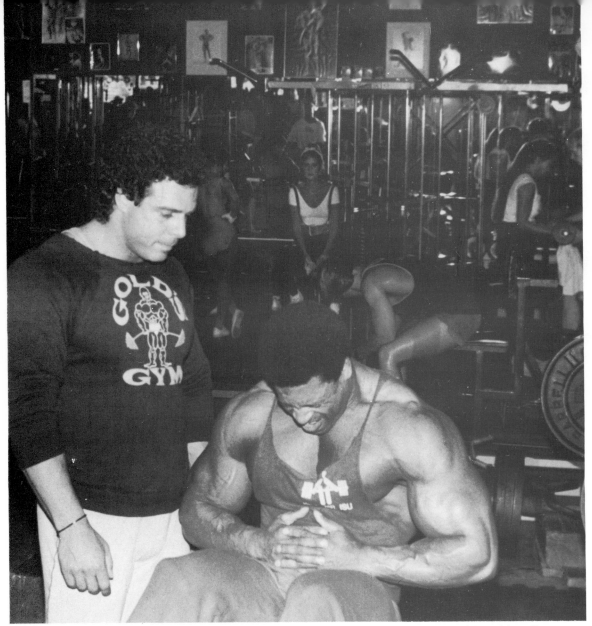

Massive Bill Grant is watched by Richard Martinelli as he goes to town on his midsection.

overtraining syndrome than other muscles. If you cannot hold back your enthusiasm, and as a result stay too long in the gym, do not be surprised if your rate of progress is zero or less.

Overtraining can make you lose ground, too. You will get smaller. Your muscles will look flat and stringy, and you'll always feel tired and run down. The answer, of course, is to control your accelerating enthusiasm. Slow down the pace and decide to make haste slowly.

Goal Setting

Once you are past the beginner's stage of bodybuilding, your progress will slow down or even stop. This is natural because you have taken your strength and development to a higher degree. Your efforts in the gym have been translated into physical fitness, strength, health, and body development. But to reach a new plateau will take even greater effort. You will have to use more weight in your exercises, added concentration, and increased intensity. It is at this juncture that the champions depart company from the less ambitious bodybuilders. While the average personalities may well continue to train, and even put in respectable workouts, those in the championship category will consciously set goals and go all out to achieve them. Goal setting is the secret of bodybuilding success. The trick, however, is to set small achievable goals and then once reached, select a new achievable goal, and so on.

It is often a good idea to select a champion bodybuilder who has a body type similar to your own. Obviously, if you are a short, narrow-shouldered, broad-hipped woman, you wouldn't select a willowy woman like Cory Everson or Anja Langer to be your role model. Neither would a tall, long-legged, broad-shouldered man choose Rich Gaspari or Tom Platz as a role model. Select someone close to your body type. That person can then be your goal target. At the turn of the century, Eugene Sandow was the hero of half the civilized world. Following him came Sig Klein, John Grimek, Steve Reeves, Reg Park, Sergio Oliva, Arnold Schwarzenegger, Lou Ferrigno, and Lee Haney. Lisa Lyon led the women's army of enthusiasts. Then came Rachel McLish, Cory Everson, Juliette Bergman, and Anja Langer. Each era has its super-star heroes and role models according to the fashion of the day.

Goal setting should be a twofold plan. The champion you select as a role model is your long-term goal. Ultimately, of course, it is within the realm of possibility that you may surpass this person's build, but for now be content to aim to achieve a comparable physique. This

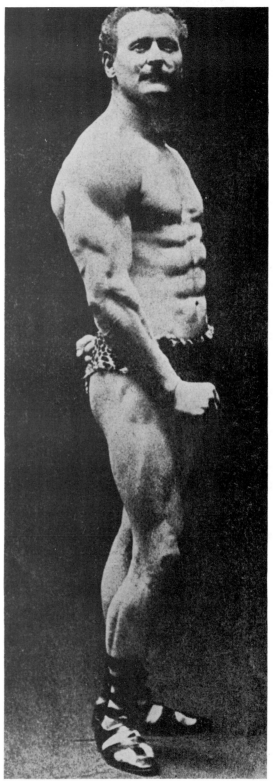

Legendary Eugene Sandow was famous for his outstanding abs.

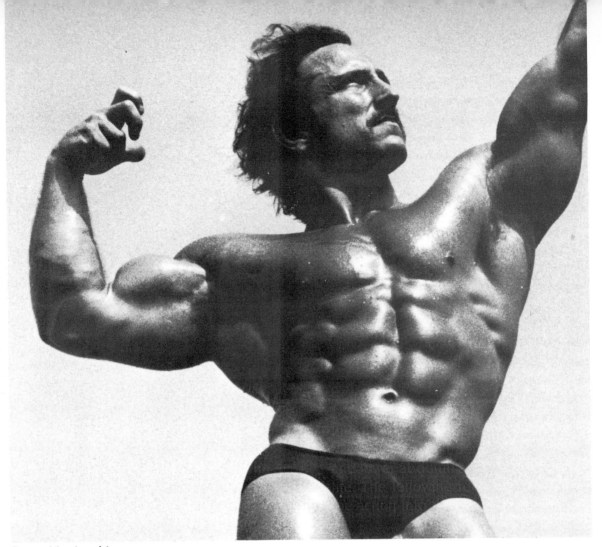

Dave Mastorakis

is no mean achievement if you have selected one of the top champions to be your hero.

You should also set short-term goals. Remember, they have to be *realistic*. As you achieve them, then set new achievable goals as mentioned earlier.

Listen to the advice of multi-time Mr. Olympia Lee Haney:

Before you think about doing reps on the bench press with 400 pounds, you have to be able to rep out with 250, 300, and 350 pounds. Don't think about winning a national title until you work at winning a city title, then state and regional competitions.

Yes, goal setting will be your passport to the ultimate physique.

Stickability

To succeed, you must have stickability. You must keep to your training. Stay with the right foods . . . in the right proportions . . . and keep up with your intensity. Perseverance in life is a key to success. Individual courage to stay on course is what gets the job done. When asked about his genius, Thomas Edison replied that it was 10 percent inspiration and 90 percent perspiration.

Do not cheat on your diet. Do not

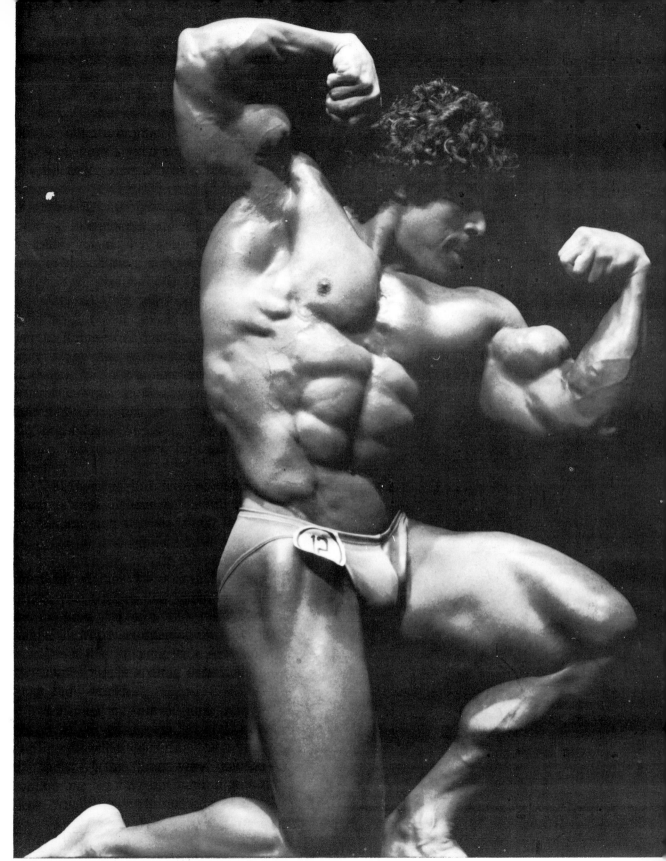

Ed Kawak shows very impressive abdominals.

miss workouts. Do not drop exercises that you know are important. Keep to your plan, come hell or high water. Stray from your goal and you will fail.

Irregular training is no good. It kills your momentum. When you miss workouts or stay out and party all night, there will be other bodybuilders who do not. And that puts them ahead of you in the rush for that trophy. Keep after your goals with relentless determination. Stick with your resolve to come out of this sport a winner. You can do it!

Concentration

People used to joke about Arnold Schwarzenegger's concentration for training. They'd say that if a bomb went off in the gym, Arnold would not even hear it if he were in the middle of a set.

Concentration means single-mindedness. It is not easy to apply yourself 100 percent. But you do become pretty good at it if you practice. To merely concentrate on completing your repetitions in a particular exercise is not enough. Your mind has to be focused on working out each specific muscle to the maximum.

For example, imagine performing wide-grip lat pulldowns on an overhead pulley machine with a workout partner. You have both completed a couple of sets of 12 reps. However, since this is a favorite exercise of your partner's, he now puts another 20 pounds of resistance on the machine and goes for another set of 12 good reps. Your ego is ruffled. You *must* also do 12 reps. You start your wide-grip pulldowns. The first three reps go well. You keep your elbows out to the side throughout the movement and you start each rep with a steady pull.

There's no heaving or jerking, no excess body movement. You are really *feeling* the stress in those lats.

Then suddenly, your next rep is hard. You are starting to fail. Determined to complete 12 reps, you now focus your mind on getting 12 reps—any way you can. In order to accomplish this, your good exercise form has deteriorated into an all-out jerk-type pulldown, instead of a smooth wide-grip elbows-back pull behind neck. You get your 12 reps, but you did it without working your lats. Instead, you solicited the lower back and the arms, giving them a second-rate workout.

Use heavy weights in your training, but not so heavy that you cannot perform the exercises correctly. Never take your concentration away from the muscle you are working just so that you can do a certain number of repetitions. If you are working the abdominals, concentrate completely on working only them. You must put your mind inside the muscle and force the action into making that muscle really feel the stimulation. If you are just concerned with lifting a weight up, then you are merely adopting a weightlifter's mentality (which is not good for a bodybuilder). Your job is to become a "feeler" and concentrate the action precisely into the muscle being worked.

Of course, there are other things that can interfere with concentration. Emotional problems are extremely distracting. Money problems and business or school dilemmas, too, can ruin your workouts. Try your best to conduct your life with reasonable care and attention so that worries are minimized. One thing's for sure: If you can't keep your concentration pinpointed on your workouts, then you are wasting your time.

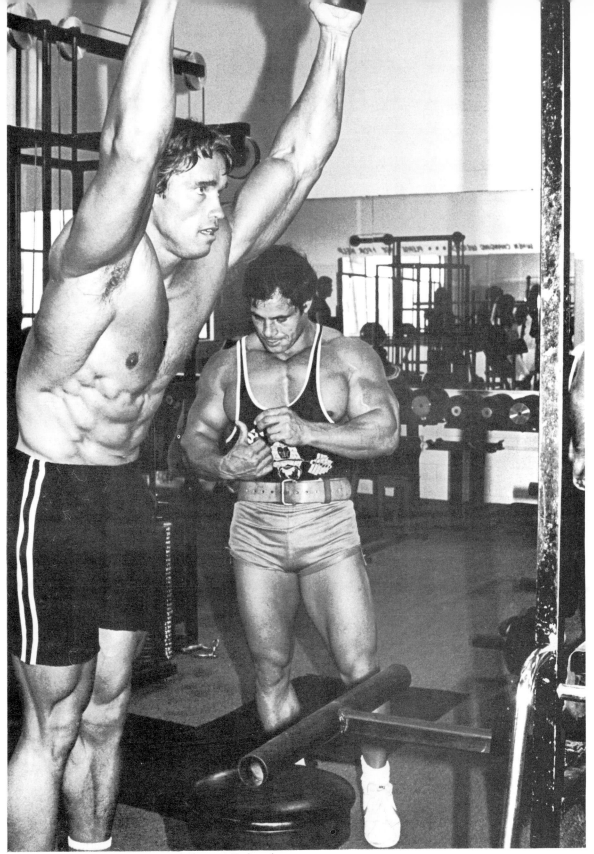

Arnold Schwarzenegger and Franco Columbu

Bodybuilding

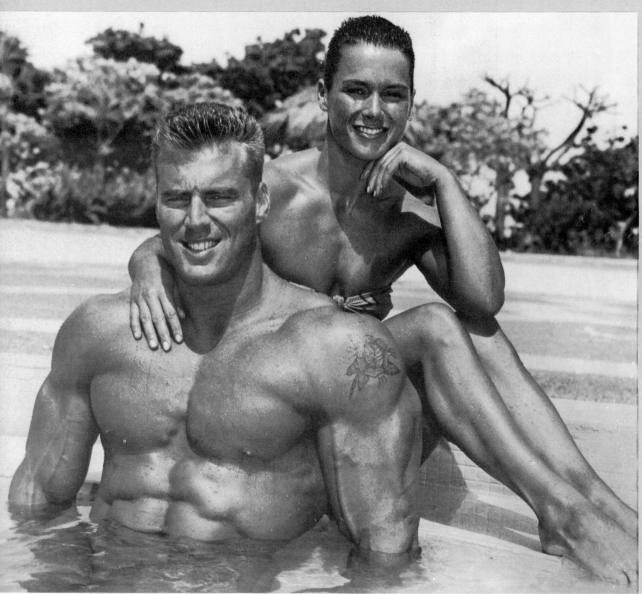

Erika Mes and Berry DeMey

Nutrition

Eating is one of the most natural things we do. Most of us, however, do it badly. Where bodybuilding is concerned, the foods we eat and the quantities we consume affect our progress in very definite ways.

Bodybuilders trying to gain weight invariably eat too little. Those wishing to lose weight frequently eat too much. But it goes deeper than that because foods are not all alike. Some foods are excellent, many are just okay, but a large amount of nutritionally deficient food is downright junk.

Let's get down to essentials. Junk foods should be avoided as much as possible. It may be difficult to avoid them altogether because frequently we have to eat in restaurants or canteens where, for the most part, food is processed and lacking in freshness. Junk food often contains huge amounts of sugar or salt. Both items are necessary in their natural form, yet we tend to overindulge in table salt and white sugar. This excessive consumption interferes with our health and energy levels. We must try and keep them out of our diets. Another demon is fat. Most of us eat entirely too much of it in the form of red meat, butter, whole milk, or deep-fried foods. Everyone should curtail fat intake, even though some is necessary for good health.

Watch what you eat whether it is a full-sized meal or a minuscule snack. The foods we eat contribute to the condition of our muscle tone, skin complexion, health, vitality, and strength, as well as the everyday functions of our bodies. If we eat junk food, then sooner or later we will start looking less than our best—and feel even worse!

The following are some of the foods and drinks that you should try to avoid.

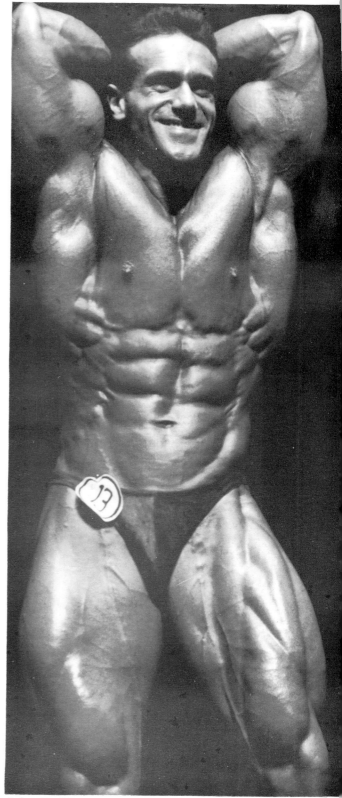

John Terilli

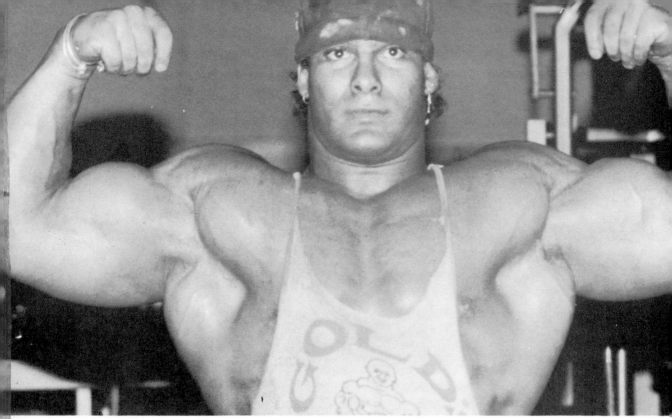

Barbarian David Paul

Do not make a regular habit of eating: canned fruit and vegetables, gravies, cream, jams and jellies, ice cream, pastries and cakes, candies and chocolates, cookies, processed cheeses, potato chips, sugar-loaded cereals, salad dressings, canned soups, crackers, pizza, smoked or processed meats, french fries, pretzels, soft drinks, artificial creams, puddings, and alcohol.

The foods we *should* eat for optimal health, vitality, and bodybuilding results include a wide variety of fruits and vegetables, milk, rice, poultry and other lean meats, whole-wheat bread, unsalted nuts, cottage cheese, raisins, salad greens, eggs, fish, yogurt, and whole grains. In my opinion, the very best foods known to man include liver, beans, rice, bananas, whole wheat, spinach, skim milk, eggs, and fish, all of which are favorites of bodybuilders.

Remember that the way in which food is cooked and prepared is important, too. Foods that are overcooked lose their nutritional value. Consume your meats and proteins lightly cooked and eat fruits and vegetables raw when at all possible. It is far healthier to grill, broil, and steam foods than deep fry them. Even boiling can cook out the goodness if the process is continued for too long. Foods should always be consumed in a state as near to the way nature produced them as possible. A whole apple is better than apple juice because of the natural fiber. Peanuts are better than peanut butter because they contain no additives.

If you are interested in making the very best bodybuilding gains, then make sure you eat the best foods. You should take your daily nutrition from the following food groups.

- *Milk* (milk, yogurt, cottage cheese, hard cheese)
- *Meats* (beef, veal, lamb, pork, fish, poultry, eggs)
- *Vegetables* (fruits, vegetables, legumes, nuts)
- *Grains* (breads, cereals)
- *Fats* (butter, margarine, oil in small amounts)

Never evaluate your foods solely by their calorie value. You must aim for the best possible return for every calorie consumed, which is why you must avoid those sugar-loaded, calorie-dense foods. Calorie-dense foods are those junky concoctions that you find in convenience stores or canteen vending machines. They are manufactured to appeal to the taste buds rather than to feed your body what it needs. Some people are so hooked on this chemically treated junk that they almost live on it. Processed foods are designed not to maximize health or satisfy your hunger and genuine nutritional needs, but to create a craving for more of the same junk food. Most packaged or canned foods are processed and considered calorie-dense. They move through your system poorly, are totally unbalanced nutritionally, and make you want to overeat.

It is true that a person who leads a moderately active life has a daily requirement of about 15 calories per pound of body weight. Generally speaking, you should eat somewhat less than this if you need to lose weight, and eat more if you desire to gain weight.

Bodybuilder Mohamed Makkawy said that in order to lose weight, "You must reduce your calories by 3,500 for every pound you wish to lose, assuming your energy output or activity level remains the same. To burn fat off your

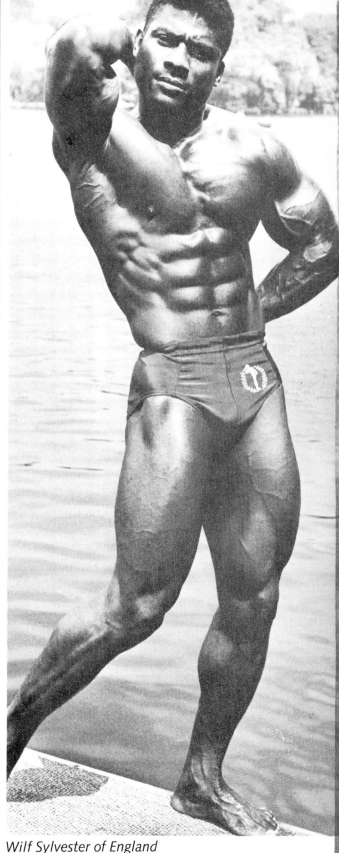

Wilf Sylvester of England

71

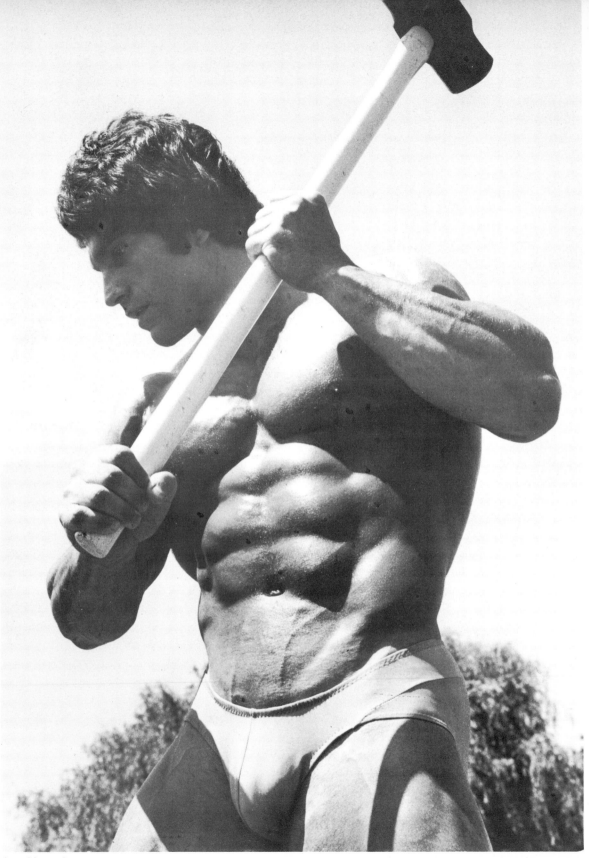

Joe Nazario

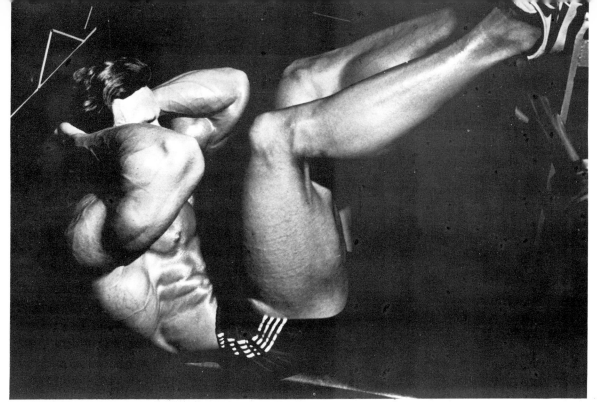

Boyer Coe does the crunch exercise.

body, you must gradually reduce your calories and increase your energy output so that you are using up more calories than you are taking in, forcing the body to use stored body fat as fuel."

The important thing to remember is that you must find the proper balance of diet and exercise that works for you through trial and error. You can reduce your overall calorie intake by just 500 calories per day to lose 3,500 per week, which translates into one pound of fat. This may not seem like much, but it is best to lose slowly when getting in shape for a bodybuilding competition. Never try to lose more than two pounds of fat per week.

To keep from getting a swollen waistline, try eating five or six small meals each day rather than three large meals, which can stretch the stomach. Also, when trying to lose weight, do not eat anything after seven o'clock at night,

since you are less active at this time and tend to store calories rather than burn them up.

British bodybuilding nutritionist Bernard Beverley said:

Of the three major elements in your diet—carbohydrate, fat, and protein—protein is the most important because it is the only thing from which your body can recreate cells and stimulate growth. The two other items are primarily needed for energy. Protein is the constructor of the body.

When you exercise, the muscle cells are broken down and it is the ingested protein that enables them to build up during rest. What some bodybuilders fail to realize is that protein is required for many vital bodily functions, including the production of blood and hormones. Your teeth, bones, and even your hair need protein. You can be sure of one thing:

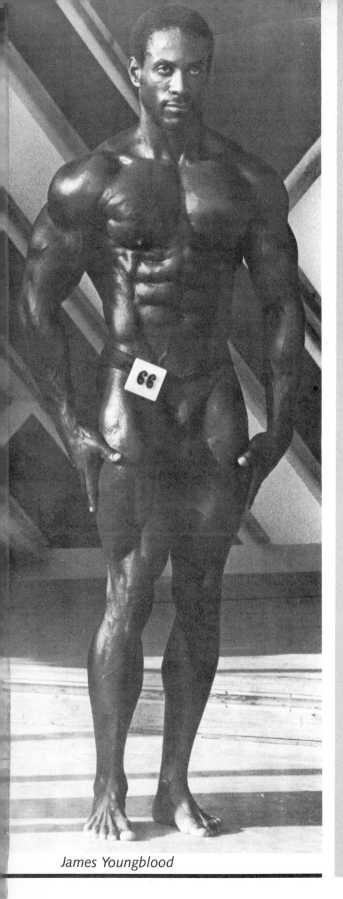

James Youngblood

The protein you eat will be utilized for body maintenance before any is allocated to increasing muscle hypertrophy.

Bernard Beverley wrote:

A bodybuilder needs ample amounts of protein over and above the survival level. In relative terms, this means 0.6 grams of protein for every pound of body weight. So a 150-pound man would need 90 grams of protein daily. While the body will grow to some extent on this amount, by a strange quirk of nature, it is far easier for the system to absorb what it needs from an abundance rather than from just enough.

In other words, if you take in more protein than you need, you'll absorb what you do need much easier. A hard-training bodybuilder would probably require about one gram of protein per pound of body weight to significantly increase muscle mass. The best protein foods include eggs, milk, organ meats (liver is excellent), red meats, poultry, fish, cheese, and nuts. If you want to count up grams, most bookstores have calorie charts and gram-counter booklets, which sell for a very modest cost.

Carbohydrates are a vital part of your diet. In fact, 60 percent of your food intake should consist of complex carbohydrates. A bodybuilder should always eat carbohydrates whenever he or she eats protein. If you do not have complex carbohydrates (vegetables, breads, cereals, rice, pasta, fruit) present with your protein, your system will convert the protein not into amino acids as it should for muscle building, but into urea, which is eliminated in your urine. You do not need great amounts of complex carbohydrates, but some are required each time you consume a high-protein food.

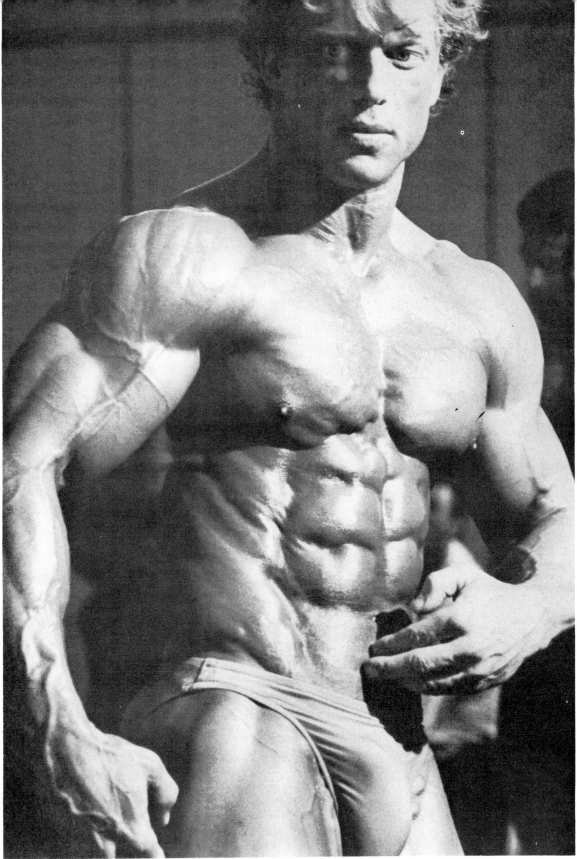

Andreas Cahling

Diets for a Fat-Free Waistline

Holland's Berry DeMey

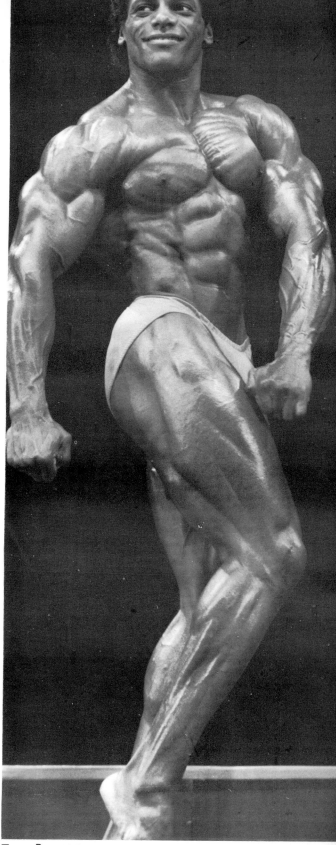

Tony Pearson

Let's assume you've decided to enter a bodybuilding contest and you know that your abs have to show up in bold relief as never before. Or perhaps you just want to look good for a special vacation in the sun. Either way, you want to maximize the look of your abdominals.

Well, here's your only alternative: You will only get results by combining a minimum of three different abdominal exercises with a progressively structured calorie-reduced food intake. The fact that I'm telling you in plain words is that if you want an outstanding, sharp-looking set of abs, you will positively *have* to diet!

First set your mind on following a sensible diet. You can do it if you really want to. Remember that the first week or so on a new diet is the hardest, but you can make this a painless experience if you reduce your calories by only minimal amounts during this early stage. Gradually, you will get used to it. Your stomach shrinks and your craving for food diminishes.

You must cut your calories, eat fewer starches, and far less fat. Learn to eat smaller amounts at every meal. You can eat up to five or six times a day if you like, but the quantity has to be controlled drastically. I must have seen scores of books and articles that claim to help people lose fat both effortlessly and painlessly. My own observations have always been that sticking to a very strict low-calorie diet is a drag, especially in those early weeks.

You must cut out all junk foods at this time more than ever. I'm well aware that friends will offer to buy you a meal, that there will be times when your co-workers are feasting on hamburgers or pizza. You'll feel so tempted to accept

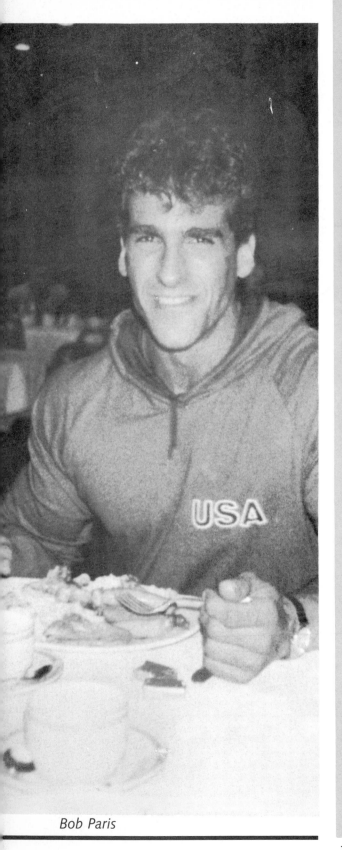

Bob Paris

just one little bite . . . but hold on. Keep that discipline intact. The craving will pass and afterwards you will be so proud that you passed up the offer. You may have had five minutes of near ecstasy chomping down the burger and fries, but think what it would do to your abdominals. It's like putting an extra blanket of fat over them!

Few things can be worse than standing on stage to compare midsections with someone who has a superb set of abs, looking like huge lumps of granite under the skin. Especially when all you have to show are a few shallow bumps under a sea of cellulite. Don't wait until the last minute to diet. You will have to allow enough time for the slimming down process, depending on how fat you are. If you are 12 pounds overweight, then six weeks is your minimum dieting time.

A diet to lose fat must still be a balanced meal plan, containing plenty of leafy green and yellow vegetables, lean, broiled meats, especially fish and poultry. High-calorie foods like potatoes, bread, and rice should still be eaten, but quantities should be carefully limited. If you are training hard, there is no need to reduce your food intake below 1,000 calories if you are a woman, or 1,500 for men. Starvation diets are neither productive nor healthy. In fact your body's natural reaction is to slow down the metabolism to the extent that your body can survive on unbelievably small amounts of nourishment. You don't lose the weight and you have defeated your purpose.

I certainly cannot list every food and its calorie content. Although it's a good idea to familiarize yourself with the approximate calorie count associated with some specific foods, it is just not practical to count every calorie. In fact, it's an im-

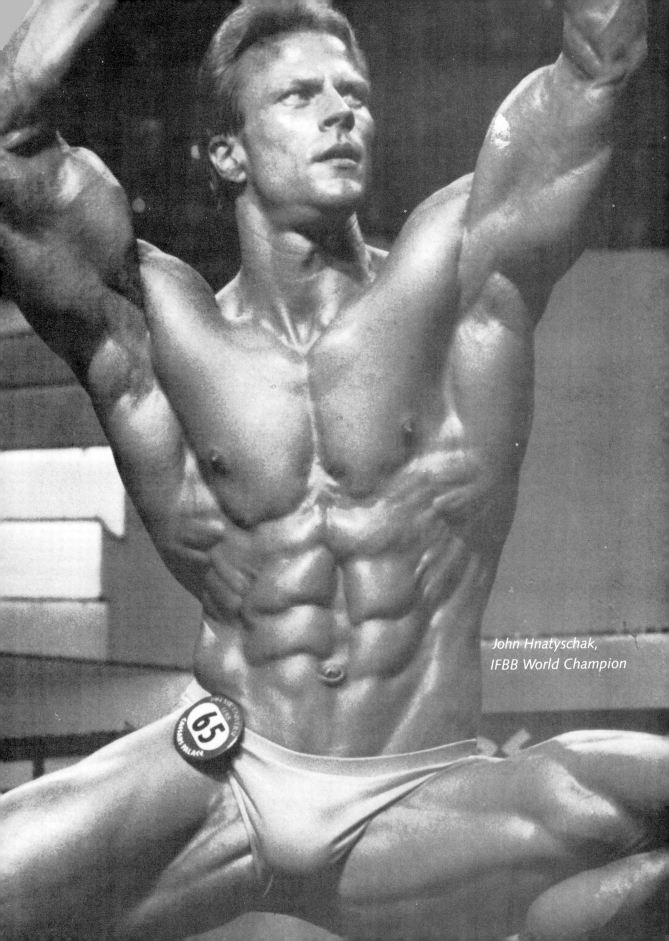

John Hnatyschak,
IFBB World Champion

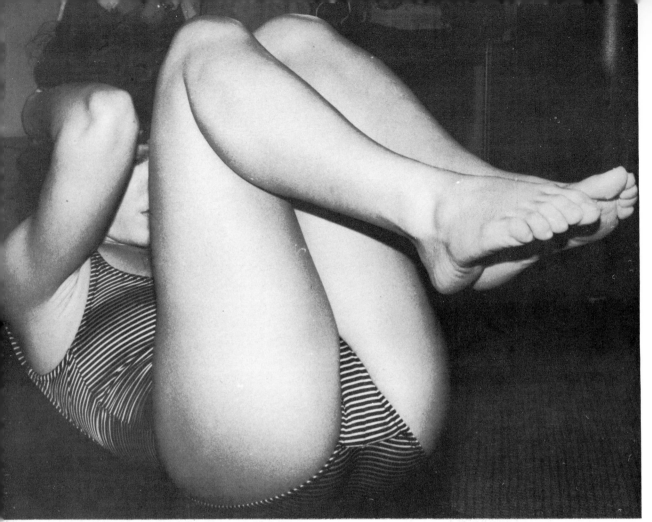

Lydia Cheng does crunches for her abs.

possible task. How can you gauge the calories in a potato? Is it a small one, a medium-size, or a big potato? You may find it helpful to buy a book that lists the calories for a variety of foods—and use it.

When defining the abdominals and trimming the waistline, you have to attack on all sides. Diet is indeed the key, but that doesn't mean you should ignore the other aspects. Work some type of aerobic activity into your day. Start with just two sessions weekly, then as you approach your target date, increase your aerobic sessions to four or even five times a week. The best activities include walking, jogging, cycling, aerobic dancing, rowing, hiking, and stationary bike work.

As for the abdominal workouts, you will develop your own favorite routines from the ones listed in this book. However, the most successful precontest routines that I ever witnessed include the use of giant sets, which is four or five different abdominal movements performed one after the other. Repeat the entire sequence three times. A typical precontest giant set follows.

Abdominal Giant Set	Reps
Hanging Knee Raise	35
Weighted Roman Chair Sit-up	25
Seated Side Twist	250
Crunch	20
Knee Tuck	50

Bodybuilders who wanted to fine tune their abs (and consequently the rest of their bodies) used to eat a diet of only meat (or fish) and water, perhaps with a few vegetables. This drastic no-carbohydrate method is now outdated. People have discovered that moderate carbohydrate intake is the answer. Today most successful male and female bodybuilders follow a low-fat, low-calorie diet, while eating plenty of complex carbohydrates, vegetables, and moderate amounts of protein.

As for supplements that help bring out muscle definition, there is a case for taking choline and inositol tablets and plenty of free-form amino acids. However, it is not a good idea to take diuretics or thyroid tablets (unless there is a specific water problem or glandular malfunction) unless specifically prescribed by a doctor.

Bodybuilding expert and writer Bill Reynolds said, "No one ever promised it would be easy to win a bodybuilding competition. Dig in and do daily aerobic sessions and diet progressively more strictly."

The following are some low-calorie diets suitable for men and women who want to cut down on their body fat while preparing for a bodybuilding contest or lose some excess weight around their midsections while performing abdominal routines. They are given in 1,000-, 1,500-, and 2,000-calorie daily plans.

Joy Nichols

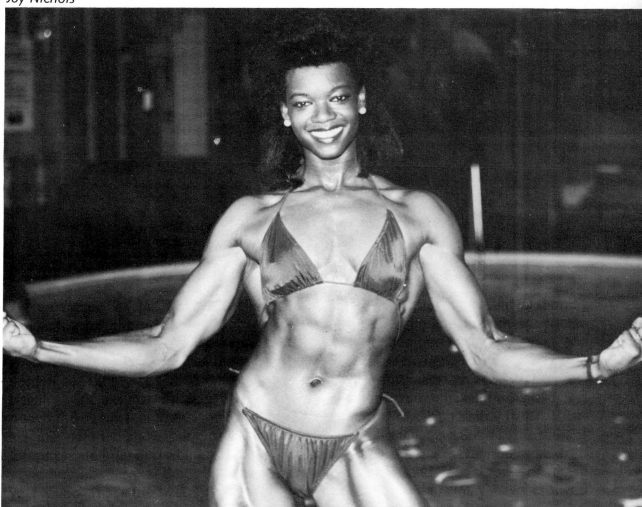

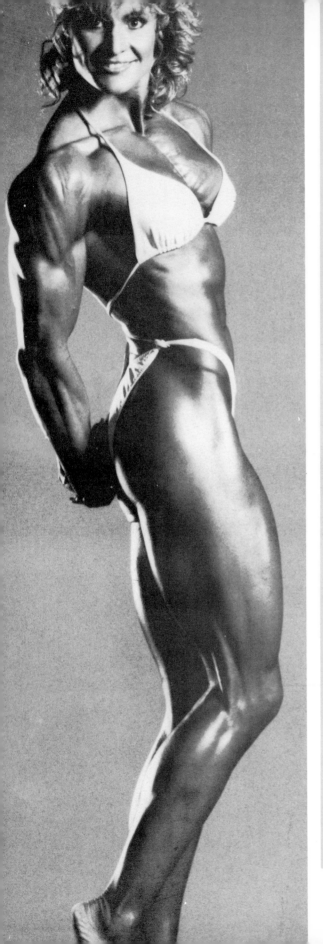

1,000-Calorie Sample Menus
Day One

Breakfast	Calories
½ cantaloupe	60
6 oz. plain yogurt	90
½ cup sliced strawberries	30
1 slice whole-wheat toast	55
coffee/tea	
Total calories	**235**

Mid-morning Snack	
1 hard-boiled egg	80
½ cup orange juice	60
Total calories	**140**

Lunch	
3 oz. sliced chicken (no skin)	120
celery and carrot sticks	20
6 cherry tomatoes	25
2 slices melba toast	30
coffee/tea	
Total calories	**195**

Mid-afternoon Snack	
1 bran muffin	85

Dinner	
3 oz. broiled halibut steak	150
⅓ cup brown rice	90
mixed salad (no dressing)	30
coffee/tea	
Total calories	**270**

Evening Snack	
½ cup skim milk	45
1 peach	40
Total calories	**85**

Corinna Everson, Ms. Olympia

Day Two

Breakfast	Calories
½ cup orange juice	60
1 poached egg	80
1 slice whole-wheat toast	55
coffee/tea	
Total calories	**195**

Mid-morning Snack	
4 oz. plain yogurt	60
½ cup blueberries	45
Total calories	**105**

Lunch	
4 oz. tuna fish (water packed)	145
6 cherry tomatoes	25
green pepper strips	20
2 slices melba toast	30
coffee/tea	
Total calories	**220**

Mid-afternoon Snack	
1 orange	70
1 slice raisin toast	65
Total calories	**135**

Dinner	
3 oz. broiled chicken	120
½ baked potato	70
mixed salad (no dressing)	30
coffee/tea	
Total calories	**220**

Evening Snack	
1 apple	70
½ cup skim milk	45
Total calories	**115**

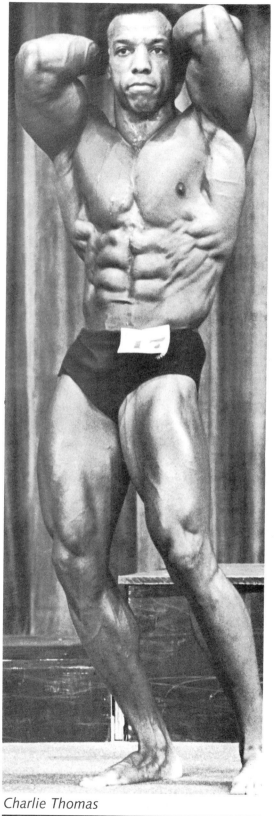

Charlie Thomas

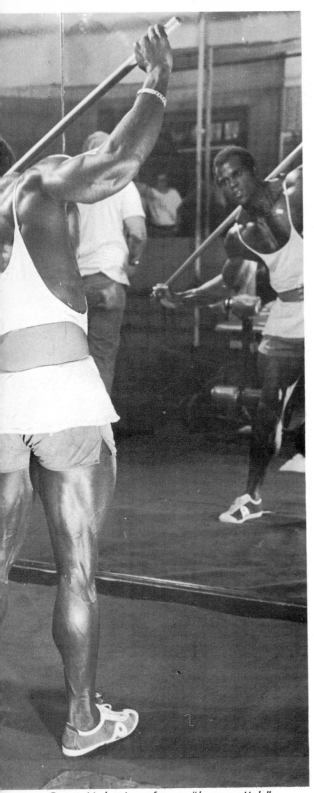

Serge Nubret performs "broomstick" twists for his waistline.

Day Three

Breakfast	Calories
½ pink grapefruit	60
omelette (2 egg whites, 1 yolk)	100
1 tsp. butter	100
1 slice whole-wheat toast	55
coffee/tea	
Total calories	**315**

Mid-morning Snack	
1 pear	80
½ cup skim milk	45
Total calories	**125**

Lunch	
½ cup cottage cheese	110
2 slices melba toast	30
coffee/tea	
Total calories	**140**

Mid-afternoon Snack	
1 cup tomato juice	45
carrot and celery sticks	20
Total calories	**65**

Dinner	
2 oz. beef liver	140
1 broiled tomato	25
½ cup steamed spinach	20
1 small potato, boiled	100
coffee/tea	
Total calories	**285**

Evening Snack	
4 oz. plain yogurt	60
½ cup diced pineapple	40
Total calories	**100**

1,500-Calorie Sample Menus
Day One

Breakfast	Calories
⅔ cup raisin bran flakes	100
½ cup 2 percent milk	60
1 banana	80
coffee/tea	
Total calories	**240**

Mid-morning Snack	
1½ oz. cashews (unsalted)	240
1 orange	70
Total calories	**310**

Lunch	
2 oz. lean roast beef	140
1 slice whole-wheat bread	55
coffee/tea	
Total calories	**195**

Mid-afternoon Snack	
2 oz. tuna fish (water packed)	75
1 slice melba toast	15
Total calories	**90**

Dinner	
4 oz. roast chicken	200
½ cup rice	110
½ cup green beans	15
½ cup carrots	25
coffee/tea	
Total calories	**350**

Evening Snack	
½ cup skim milk	45
1 slice whole-wheat bread	55
1 apple	70
Total calories	**170**

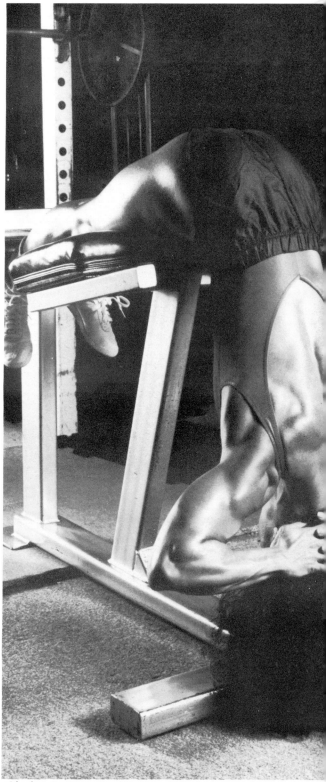

Gladys Portugues does a prone hyperextension for her lower back.

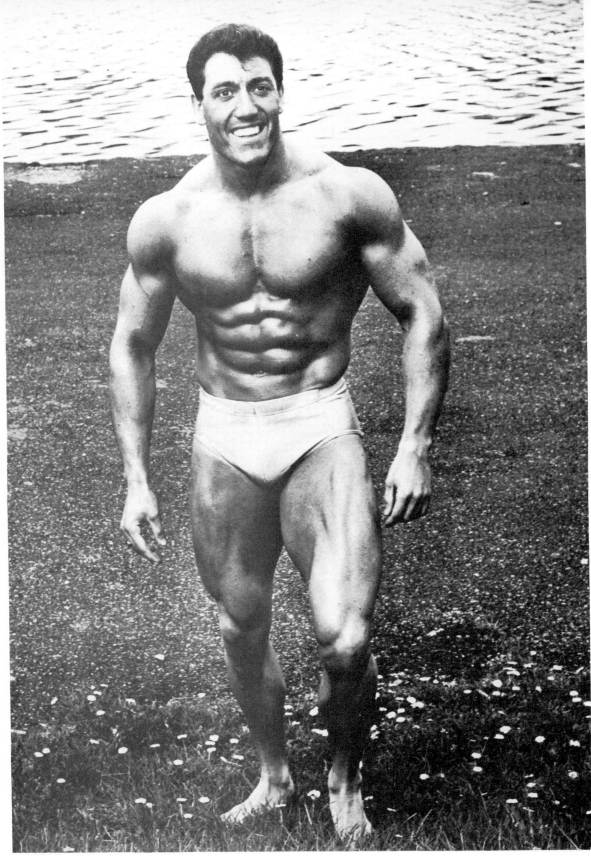

Roy Perrott

Day Two

Breakfast	Calories
½ cup orange juice	60
2 slices whole-wheat toast	110
2 oz. cheddar	
cheese (broiled on toast)	220
2 slices tomato	10
coffee/tea	
Total calories	**400**

Mid-morning Snack	
6 dried apricots	80
½ cup 2 percent milk	60
Total calories	**140**

Lunch	
3 oz. canned shrimp	75
1 stalk celery, chopped	10
1 tsp. mayonnaise	100
2 slices melba toast	30
coffee/tea	
Total calories	**215**

Mid-afternoon Snack	
1 tbsp. peanut butter	95
1 slice whole-wheat bread	55
Total calories	**150**

Dinner	
4 oz. lean ground beef patty,	
broiled	250
1 baked potato	140
mixed salad (no dressing)	30
coffee/tea	
Total calories	**420**

Evening Snack	
1 bran muffin	85
½ cup skim milk	45
Total calories	**130**

Mary Roberts

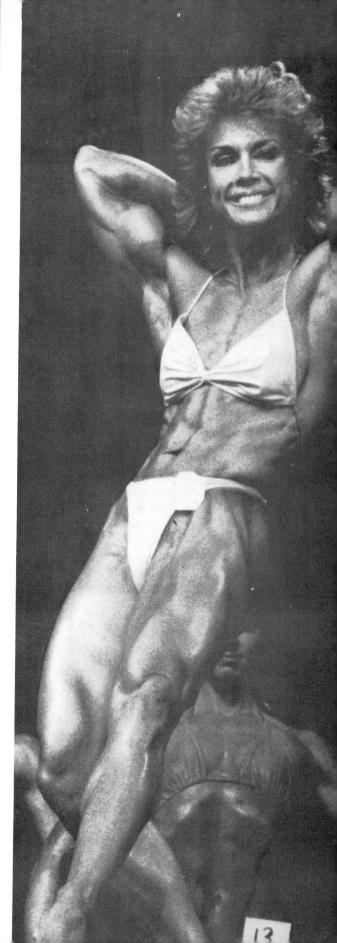

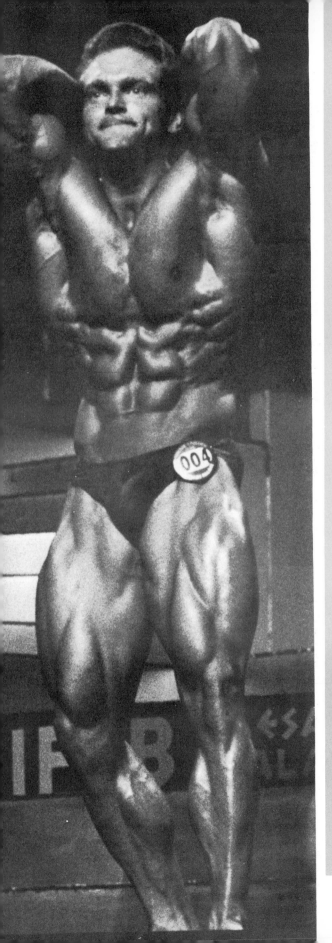

Day Three

Breakfast	Calories
½ cup pineapple juice	70
1 boiled egg	80
2 slices whole-wheat toast	110
coffee/tea	
Total calories	**260**

Mid-morning Snack	
2 slices crisp bread	90
1 wedge honeydew melon	50
½ cup skim milk	45
Total calories	**185**

Lunch	
1 cup tomato soup	90
1 oz. whole-wheat crackers	110
2 oz. Swiss cheese	200
coffee/tea	
Total calories	**400**

Mid-afternoon Snack	
1 banana	80
½ cup 2 percent milk	60
Total calories	**140**

Dinner	
4 oz. broiled sole	180
½ cup steamed broccoli	20
1 grilled tomato	25
1 baked potato	140
1 tsp. butter	100
coffee/tea	
Total calories	**445**

Evening Snack	
1 hard-boiled egg	80
1 orange	70
Total calories	**150**

Calvin Nyulli of Canada

2,000-Calorie Sample Menus
Day One

Breakfast	Calories
1 cup tomato juice	45
2 eggs, scrambled	160
1 tsp. butter	100
2 slices whole-wheat toast	110
coffee/tea	
Total calories	**415**

Mid-morning Snack	
1 apple	70
½ cup 2 percent milk	60
Total calories	**130**

Lunch	
2 oz. broiled flounder	115
1 tsp. butter	100
1 slice whole-wheat bread	55
½ cup 2 percent milk	60
coffee/tea	
Total calories	**330**

Mid-afternoon Snack	
2 oz. almonds (unsalted)	340
1 orange	70
Total calories	**410**

Dinner	
4 oz. roast turkey	200
½ cup peas	60
½ cup carrots	25
2 boiled potatoes	210
coffee/tea	
Total calories	**495**

Evening Snack	
1 cup 2 percent milk (mixed with 1 tbsp. milk-and-egg protein powder)	175
1 banana	80
Total calories	**255**

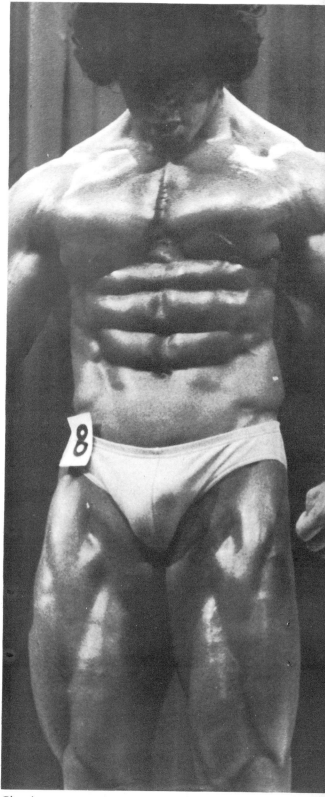

Check out Ed Kawak's super-defined abs!

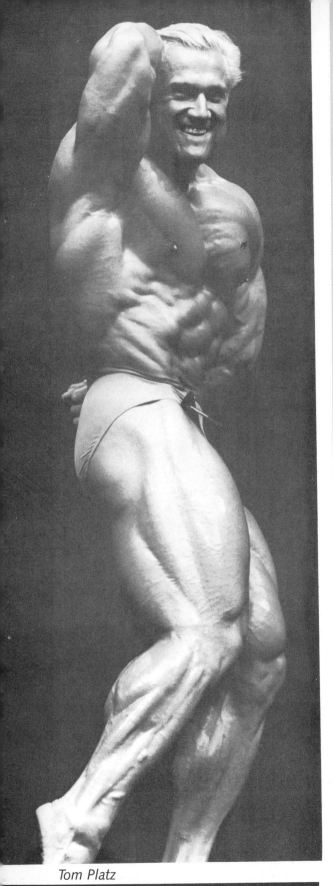

Tom Platz

Day Two

Breakfast	Calories
½ cup orange juice	60
1 cup Cream of Wheat	135
2 slices whole-wheat toast	110
½ cup 2 percent milk	60
1 banana	80
coffee/tea	
Total calories	**445**

Mid-morning Snack	
1 oz. Muenster cheese	110
3 cherry tomatoes	12
4 slices melba toast	60
Total calories	**182**

Lunch	
4 oz. sliced roast beef	200
2 slices whole-wheat bread	110
lettuce and tomato	15
1 orange	70
1 cup 2 percent milk	120
coffee/tea	
Total calories	**515**

Mid-afternoon Snack	
1 cup 2 percent milk (mixed with 2 tbsp. milk-and-egg protein powder)	220
¼ cup applesauce	60
½ banana	40
Total calories	**320**

Dinner	
2-egg Spanish omelette	180
½ cup steamed zucchini	15
1 baked potato	140
1 tsp. butter	100
coffee/tea	
Total calories	**435**

Evening Snack	
½ cup bran flakes	55
½ cup 2 percent milk	60
Total calories	**115**

Day Three

Breakfast

	Calories
1 cup oatmeal	130
½ oz. raisins	80
½ apple, chopped	35
1 slice whole-wheat toast	55
1 cup 2 percent milk	120
coffee/tea	
Total calories	**420**

Mid-morning Snack

2 hard-boiled eggs	160
2 slices melba toast	30
1 peach	40
Total calories	**230**

Lunch

2 tbsp. peanut butter	190
2 slices whole-wheat bread	110
1 cup orange juice	120
coffee/tea	
Total calories	**420**

Mid-afternoon Snack

2 oz. cheddar cheese	220
1 bran muffin	85
Total calories	**305**

Dinner

4 oz. lean broiled sirloin steak	235
½ cup green beans	15
½ cup carrots	25
1 baked potato	140
1 tsp. butter	100
coffee/tea	
Total calories	**515**

Evening Snack

6 oz. yogurt	90
½ cup sliced strawberries	30
Total calories	**120**

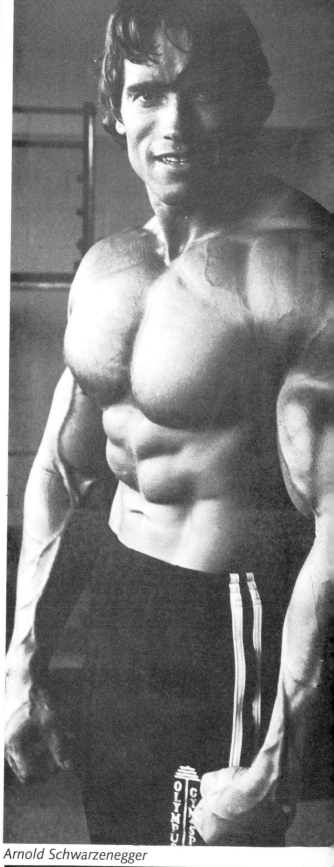

Arnold Schwarzenegger

Routines

Steve Davis

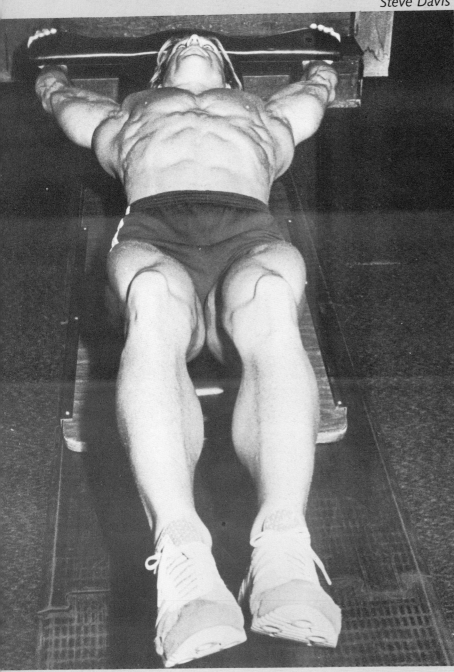

of

the

Champions

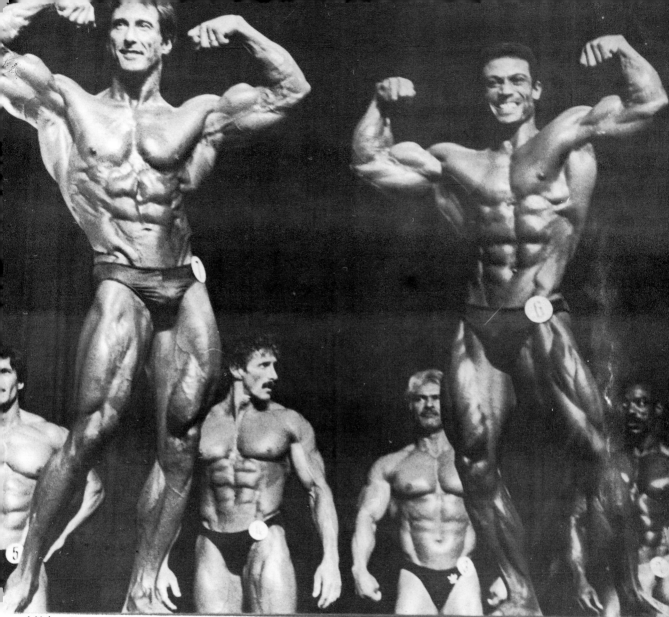

Midsection magnificence is evident in both Frank Zane and Mohamed Makkawy.

I remember Britain's Reg Park telling me that he only did direct abdominal work a few weeks prior to entering a contest. He believed that the midsection got plenty of work from overall training with weights. There are some bodybuilders who still only train their abs just before a show, but most of the top physique men and women of today work their abs several times a week all year round. That's the best way to keep them in top shape.

This chapter is devoted to showing how the champions train their abdominals. Remember that these men and women are champions. It may have taken them many years to reach the stage that they have currently achieved. Also, it is important to keep in mind that routines are always changing. Some of the champs will still be using exactly the same exercises, sets, and reps shown on these pages, but others may have changed their ab-training routines entirely.

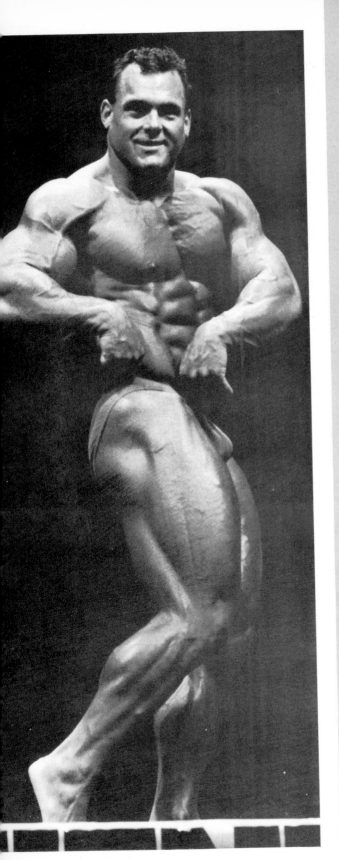

Tim Belknap

Tim hails originally from Illinois, and he won the 1981 Mr. America title. This is considered a great accomplishment for Tim because because he is a diabetic, which requires him to adjust his diet and exercise plans according to specific demands. Tim weighed less than 100 pounds when he started bodybuilding with weights. At his peak power, Tim could squat with over 700 pounds and bench press over 500. In the off season, Tim would always be huge, yet still muscular, but as a contest deadline approached he would totally transform his appearance. For the last two or three weeks, he would adhere to a 900-calorie daily diet. Tim's muscle definition would pop out like magic. His skin would change him from white to deep tan and his hair would turn blonder. Soon his totally ripped physique would be on stage and ready for one-on-one competition.

Abdominal Routine

	Sets	Reps
Crunch	5	× 20–30
Cable Leg Raise	5	× 25–30
Side Bend	5	× 30–50

Tim Belknap

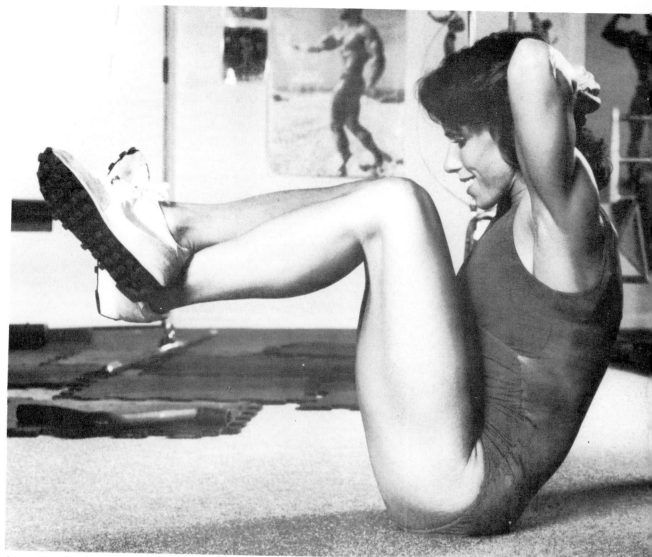

Lynn Conkwright performs her own kind of tummy training.

Lynn Conkwright

Lynn was an all-round Virginia Beach state champ in gymnastics. She did her first weight workout at the gym in her university, to develop strength for her gymnastics moves, but she soon discovered that she had what it takes to be a top bodybuilder. She began sprouting muscles all over. In 1981, she entered and won the World Women's Professional World Championships and the World Couples Championships (teamed with Chris Dickerson). She has also placed in the top three in the Ms. Olympia contest.

Abdominal Routine

	Sets	Reps
Wall Crunch (feet straight up against wall)	3	× 20–25
Hanging Leg Raise	3	× 15–20
Jackknife Crunch	3	× 20–25
Cable Crunch	3	× 20–25
Seated Twist	3	× 25–30

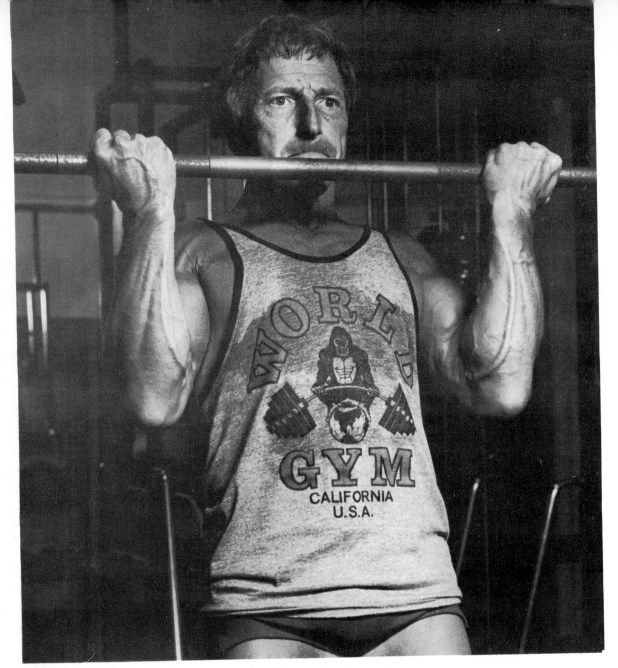

Ed Guiliani

Ed Guiliani

Originally from New York, Ed has won both the Western and Eastern Mr. America titles in addition to class wins in the Mr. America and Mr. U.S.A. with Zabo Kozewski. Ed manages the new World Gym in Venice, California. He always finishes his workouts with his waist routine, and like Zabo, he trains his abs by the clock rather than by counting the repetitions. Ed is one of the most likeable men in the sport of bodybuilding.

Abdominal Routine	Reps
Roman Chair Sit-up (upper abs)	20 minutes (about 500 reps)
Knee Tuck (lower abs)	20 minutes (about 650 reps)

Tom Platz

He's the golden boy of body-building, loved by all in the iron game. His first big win was the IFBB World Championships in 1978. Ever since then, Tom has competed many times in the pro ranks, invariably placing in the prestigious Mr. Olympia contest. Tom is recognized as being one of the hardest trainers in the world. He seldom stops a set before complete muscle failure occurs.

Abdominal Routine

	Sets	Reps
Roman Chair Sit-up	4	× to failure
Incline Twist	4	× to failure
Side Crunch	4	× to failure

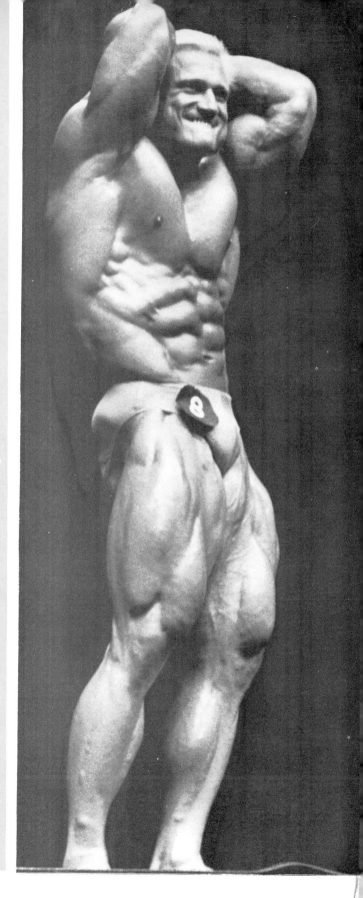

Tom Platz

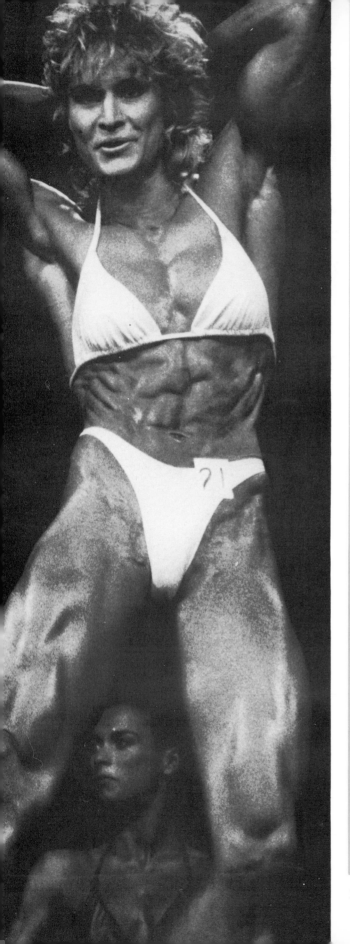

Corinna Everson

There's little doubt that Cory Everson is one of the super female bodybuilders of this decade. Even the people against whom she competes admit that her body is undeniably one of the most incredible physiques in the world. She has already won three consecutive Ms. Olympia titles and doubtless if she chooses to continue to compete, there will be more. With husband Jeff (who is also a bodybuilder of note) to help plan her workout routines and encourage her, Cory has been known to perform grueling amounts of exercises. She has done up to 30 sets per body part when training for a contest.

Abdominal Routine

	Sets	Reps
Crunch	3	× maximum
Bent-knee Leg Raise	3	× maximum
Seated Knee Raise	3	× maximum

Corinna Everson

Mohamed Makkawy

He won the 1976 Mr. Universe contest (beating out Danny Padilla) and subsequently turned pro. Then he entered the IFBB grand prix circuit and the Mr. Olympia contest. Mohamed won numerous grand prix titles and has now settled down in Toronto, Canada, where he works for multi-gym owner Ken Wheeler.

Abdominal Routine

	Sets	Reps
Crunch	3	× 12–15
Hanging Knee Raise	3	× 15–20
Seated Twist	3	× 200

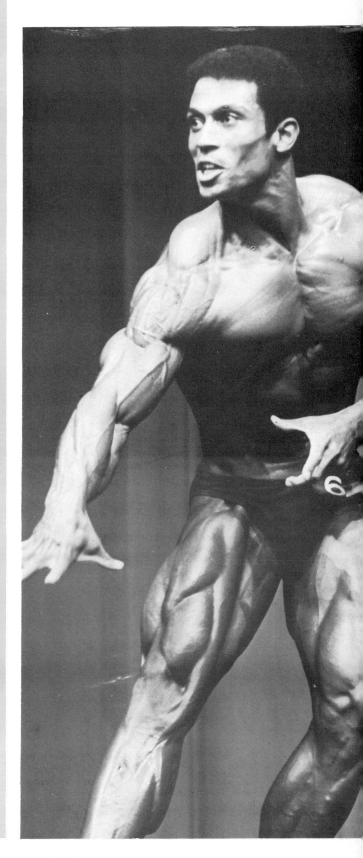

Mohamed Makkawy

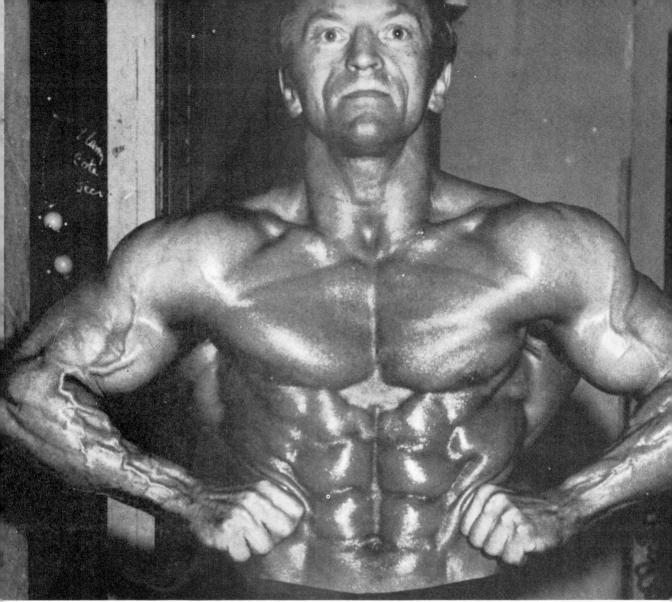

Pierre Vandensteen

Pierre Vandensteen

Pierre is now over 50 years old, but he still trains almost daily in his native Belgium. He has won the Mr. Europe and Mr. International contests as well as his height class in the Mr. Universe competition. He is known as a hardcore trainer and always believed in performing at least 25–30 sets per muscle group, three times per week to get the best results. Today this style of training is considered excessive. Most bodybuilders seem to get best results from training each muscle group twice weekly using a system of 10–15 sets per body part.

Abdominal Routine

	Sets	Reps
Roman Chair Sit-up	1	× 200
Hanging Leg Raise (twisting)	2	× 25–30
Incline Sit-up (50-lb. plate behind neck)	1	× 50
Twisting Knee Raise	2	× 100

Clare Furr

Clare Furr hails from the town of Greenwood, Mississippi. She was introduced to weight training by a friend while she was still in high school and she loved it from day one. At 5 feet 4½ inches, she has placed second in the IFBB Ms. Olympia contest to Cory Everson in 1986. She hopes one day to win the title.

Abdominal Routine

	Sets	Reps
Hanging Leg Raise (weighted)	6	× 6–10
Seated Knee Raise	5	× 6–10
Crunch	1	× 200
Twisting Crunch	1	× 100

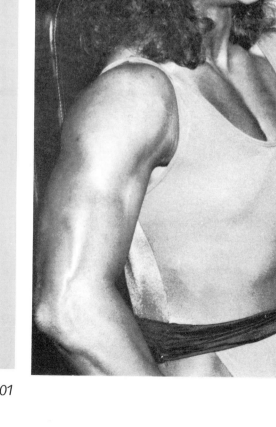

Clare Furr makes a muscle for Trent Mitchell.

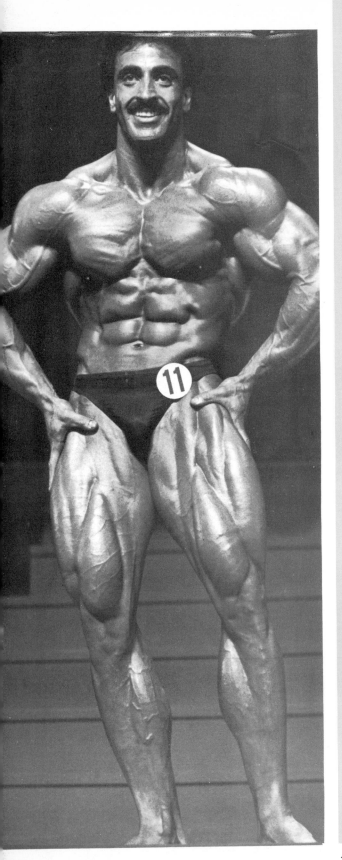

Samir Bannout

Born in Lebanon, Samir, as a young boy, moved first to England and then to the United States. He won the 1983 Mr. Olympia contest in Germany and is said to possess one of the most well-proportioned physiques in the world. Early on, Samir found difficulty in getting his abdominals to look ultra-ripped at contest time, but eventually he overcame the problem. Today he's always 100 percent in shape at contest time.

Abdominal Routine

	Sets	Reps
Roman Chair Sit-up (with weight)	4	× 25
Hanging Leg Raise	4	× 25
Intercostal Crunch (pulley machine)	4	× 30

Samir Bannout

Roy Callender

Roy is originally from the island of Barbados. He subsequently moved to England, where he lived for ten years, and then to Montreal, Canada. Currently, he owns his own gym back in his native Barbados. He still competes occasionally on the IFBB pro circuit. Roy trains each body part every three days, and he splits his routines so that he works three days without pause before taking a rest. He takes two days off after the third training day. However, he does train his abs every day to keep the muscles in peak definition. Roy doesn't usually count the number of sets he performs, choosing to work more by instinct.

Abdominal Routine

	Sets		Reps
Roman Chair Sit-up	2–4	×	30–50
Bench Leg Raise	2–4	×	50–100
Crunch	2–4	×	25–30

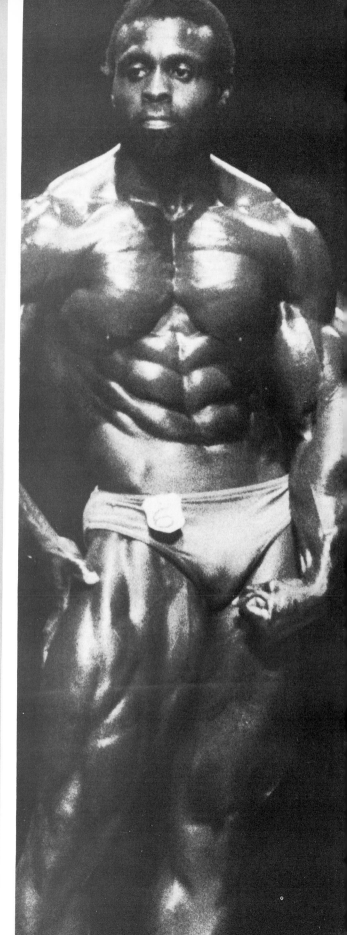

Roy Callender

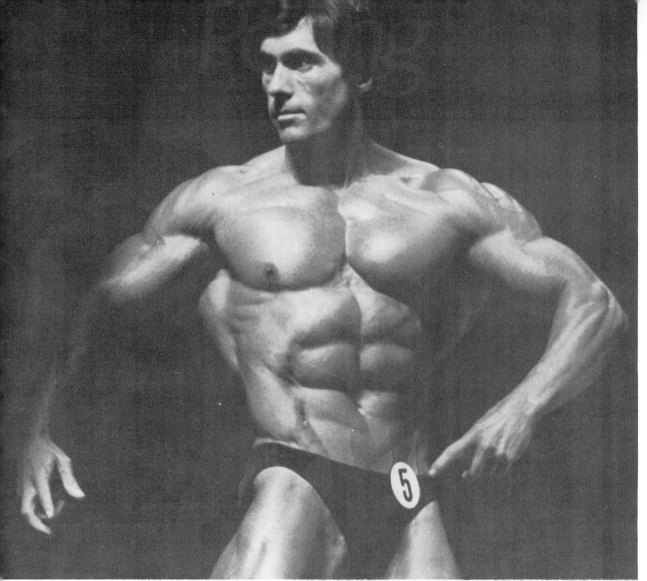

Jacques Neuville

Jacques Neuville

Jacques is on the IFBB pro circuit, but he already made an impression well before turning professional. He has won the Mr. France and the Mr. Universe titles (IFBB World Championships). He is generally considered to have the best abdominal development in pro bodybuilding. Jacques feels that he is carrying on the French tradition of leading the world in abdominal development. In his younger years, he trained his abs so hard that they actually were his most developed muscles. Currently, he performs giant sets (groups of 4–6 exercises done consecutively without a rest until the complete giant set is completed). Jacques trains his abs first in his workout when he has the most energy and enthusiasm.

Abdominal Routine

	Sets	Reps
Roman Chair Sit-up	4	× 25–30
Bench Leg Raise	4	× 25–30
Rope Crunch	4	× 25–30
Seated Twist	4	× 50

Carla Dunlap

In Carla's home state of New Jersey, she majored in commercial art at the Newark Arts High School. During her school years, she was a speed swimmer and competed in synchronized swimming. After graduating, she continued with synchronized swimming and moved to Texas, where she won the Junior National Indoor Championships. Then she took up bodybuilding.

Weight training ultimately gave Carla Dunlap an additional ten pounds, and she competed at 125 pounds body weight. She became a world champion and a couples world champion (with bodybuilder Tony Pearson). Carla trains on a three-days-on one-day-off system.

Abdominal Routine

	Sets	Reps
Seated Twist	3–4	× 50
Crunch	3–4	× 50
Hanging Leg Raise (lower abs)	4	× 50
Roman Chair Sit-up (upper abs)	4	× 50

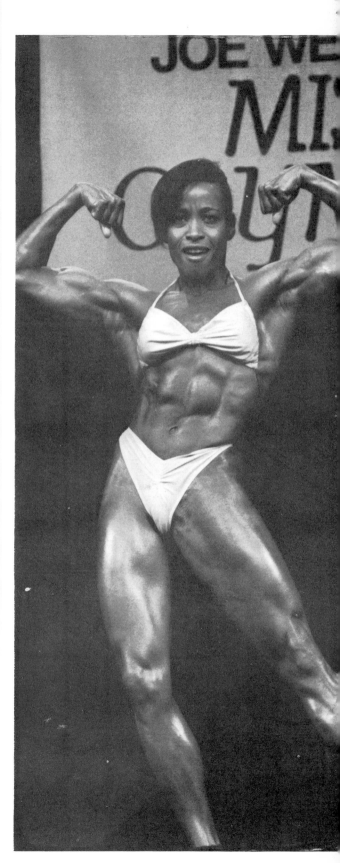

Carla Dunlap

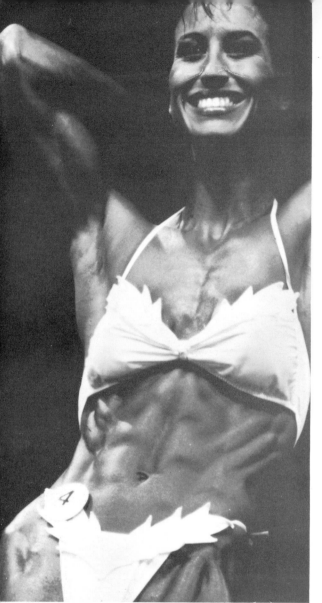

Rachel McLish

Still one of the most popular women bodybuilders in the world, Rachel is now in great demand for commercials, television, and films. In her early competitions, Rachel earned herself two Ms. Olympia titles and also top honors in U.S. bodybuilding and women's world championships. Rachel has a unique way of training for a bodybuilder. She follows a complete program of stretching, aerobics, and weight training and is very adept at many gymnastic movements.

Abdominal Routine

	Sets		Reps
Hanging Knee Raise	3	×	25
Roman Chair Sit-up (twisting)	3	×	50
Knee Tuck	5	×	50–100

Rachel McLish

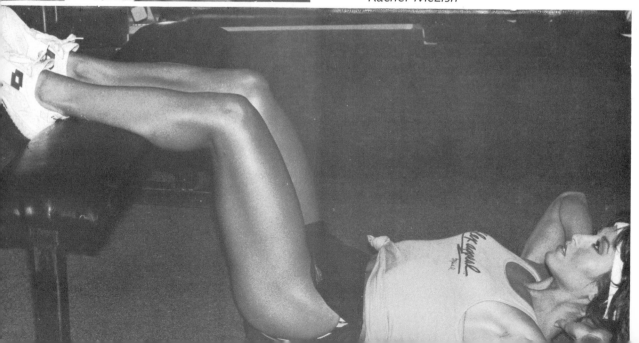

Tommy Terwillinger

This man takes his abdominal training very seriously. Tommy is a New Yorker who has steadily worked his way up the ladder of success. He is now placing well in contests on the IFBB pro circuit. He trains his abdominals two days in a row followed by one day of rest, alternating between two completely different routines.

Abdominal Routine One

	Sets	Reps
Bench Crunch (with 25-lb. plate)	4 ×	30–50
Pulley Crunch (50–100 lbs.)	3 ×	20–35
One-arm Cable Crunch (with 50 lbs., right arm to left knee and vice versa)	3 ×	25
Side Twist	3 ×	100

Abdominal Routine Two

	Sets	Reps
Bench Crunch (with legs extended straight up against bench, hands behind head)	4 ×	50
Hanging Leg Raise (lift feet as high as possible, raising hips)	3 ×	20
Supine Side Raise (with back on bench, raise legs straight upwards, then rotate sideward, right and left)	3 ×	25

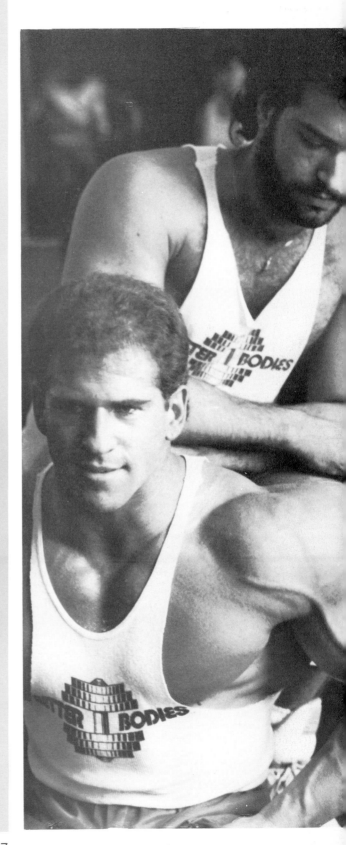

Tommy Terwillinger sits in front of Brian Moss.

Posing

Mohamed Makkawy and Frank Zane

the Abdominals

There are special high-intensity lights used to illuminate the muscles of bodybuilders on stage during a contest. Years ago, only a single overhead light was set above a posing platform. Of course, this single source of light was good for showing the pectoral, abdominal, and arm muscles, but an overhead light source does very little for the thighs, and even less for the calves, unless you happen to turn your back to the audience and rise upwards on your toes. Overhead lighting has other drawbacks as well. It's not easy to recognize who's up on stage. The eyes become mere dark pockets of shadow.

In the early seventies, lighting techniques for most bodybuilding contests changed. Various side lights and even floor lights were introduced so the judges and audiences could hardly *see* the bodybuilders on stage, even the color of their eyes. Occasionally, especially when a major contest is being filmed for television, the lighting is not carefully planned. If too much front lighting is used, everyone on stage looks flat. The best lighting I ever saw at a show was at Albert Busek's Mr. Olympia contest in Munich, Germany. Each contestant was made to look his best because of the perfectly balanced network of lights from overhead, the floor, and both sides.

From the moment you step on stage, you should be familiar with the position of the lights and how they affect your appearance. There are three different situations that you should be aware of:

1. When you are posing individually on the rostrum.
2. When you are being compared to other contestants in front of the judges.

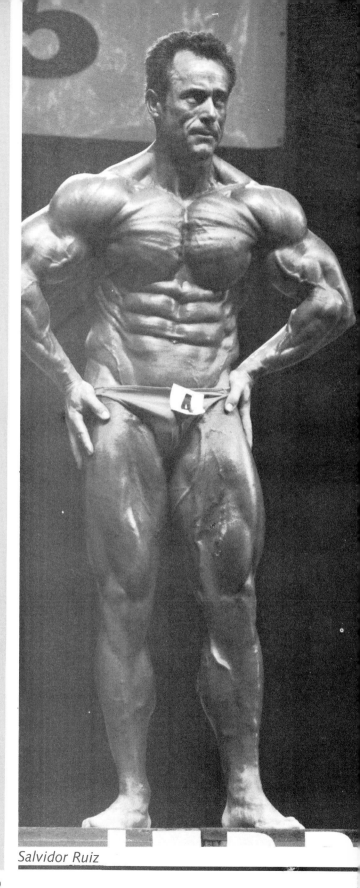

Salvidor Ruiz

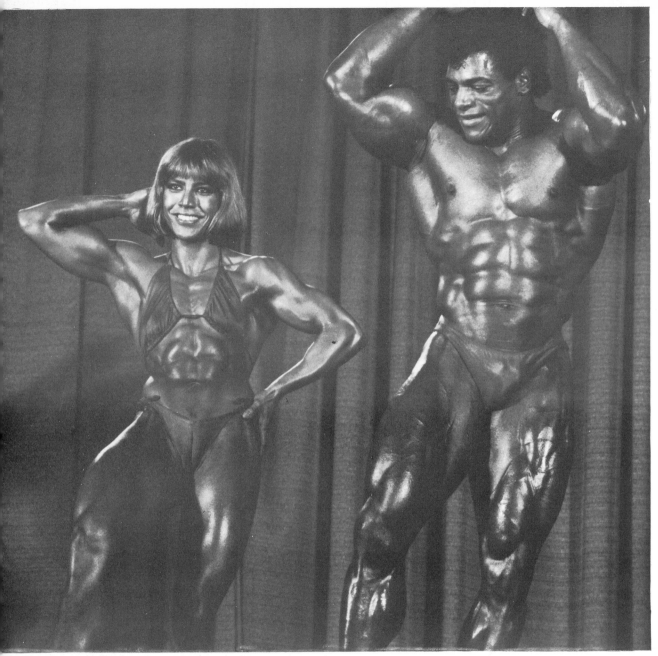

Juliette Bergman and Tony Pearson

3. When you are standing at the back of the stage while others are being compared.

In each instance, you are likely to be assessed by the judges. They will make decisions about you even when they are supposed to be appraising someone else. Accordingly, whenever you are standing on stage waiting for your turn, make sure that your abdominals are tensed. If you don't tense them, then the person next to you will, and he or she will look that much better. The same, of

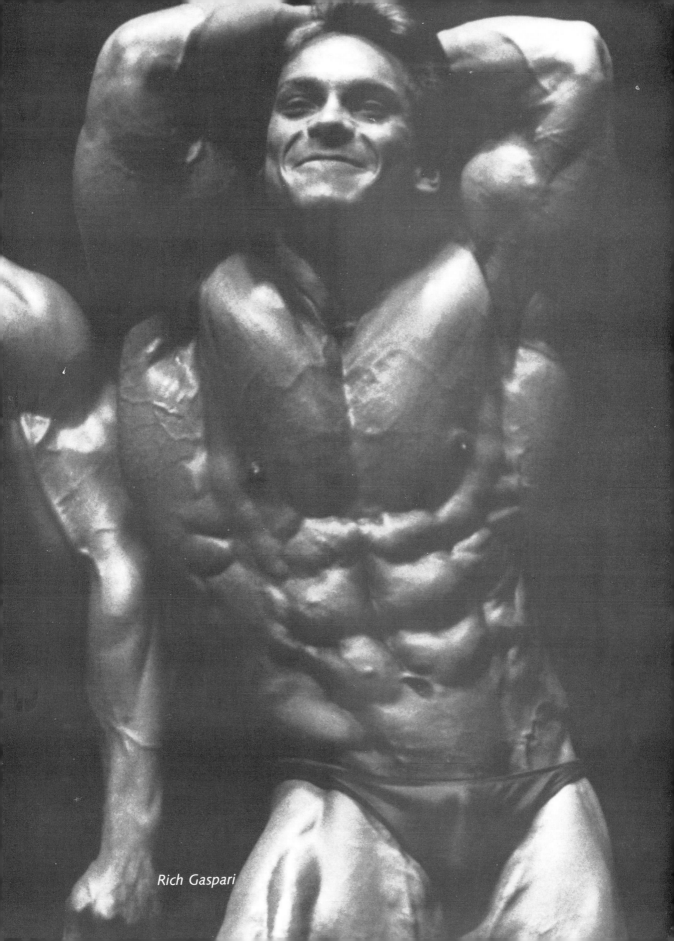

Rich Gaspari

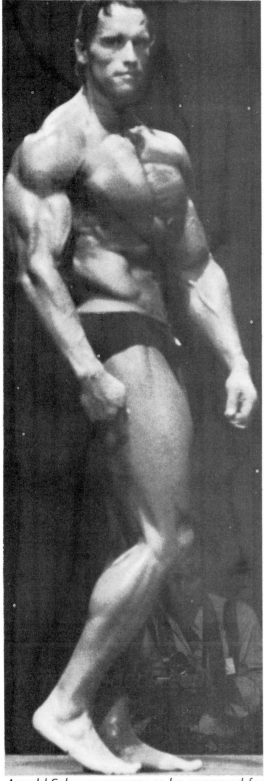

Arnold Schwarzenegger as he appeared for his last Mr. Olympia contest in Australia.

course, goes for the thighs. Relaxed thighs, like a relaxed midsection, merely look smooth and undistinguished, yet when either are tensed they can rivet the attention of the judges.

When you are on stage and in position, either in a lineup or on a posing rostrum, quickly look down at your abdominals and check that the overhead lights are hitting the upper edge of each ridge of abdominal muscle. Adapt your position quickly and never look down again. Nothing looks worse than to see bodybuilders with their heads tilted forward checking that their muscles are in the right light. Sometimes I think the bodybuilder is checking that his or her muscles are still there! Whatever the case, when you enter a contest, you should be developed enough to have confidence in your appearance. If suddenly you feel alone on stage, drained of confidence, to the extent that you have to keep checking your pecs and abs, then you are in trouble. Always hold your head up high. Resist the urge to look down. Smile confidently and show the fact that you are proud of your body.

Many bodybuilders have stated that the tedious precontest judging comparisons and stage procedures before the evening show are the most physically demanding activities possible.

"It is worse than the training," said Arnold Schwarzenegger who, during his last Mr. Olympia win in Australia, was only a heartbeat away from total exhaustion during the judging process. But he endured the ordeal and never gave in. Although he was cramping, sweating, and trembling with the effort of "keeping tight," the smile never left his face.

You must practice and actually train for the precontest judging part of a show.

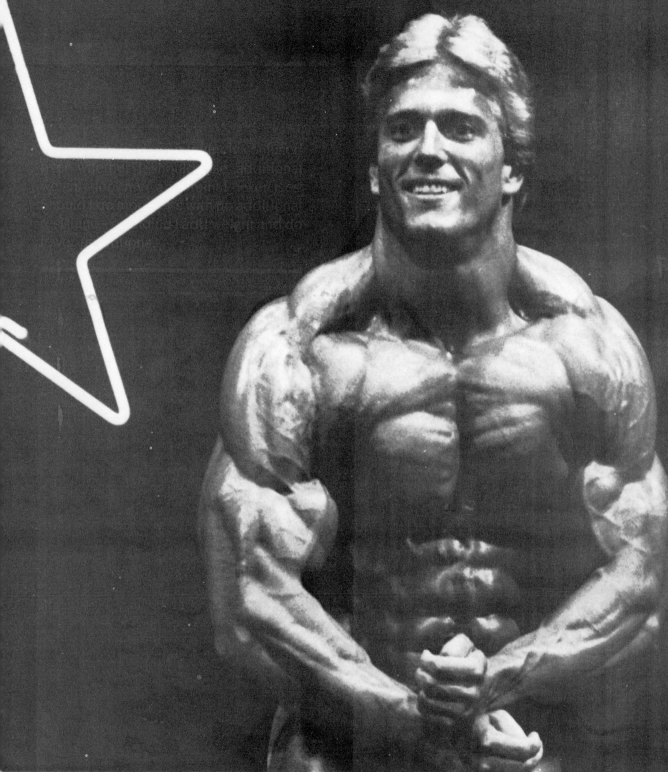

Joe Meeko

The fact is you may have to stand for 30 minutes or more with your muscles tensed—shoulders and lats out, thighs flexed, and abs tight. Beginners can do this for no more than 30 seconds, so practice as much as you possibly can.

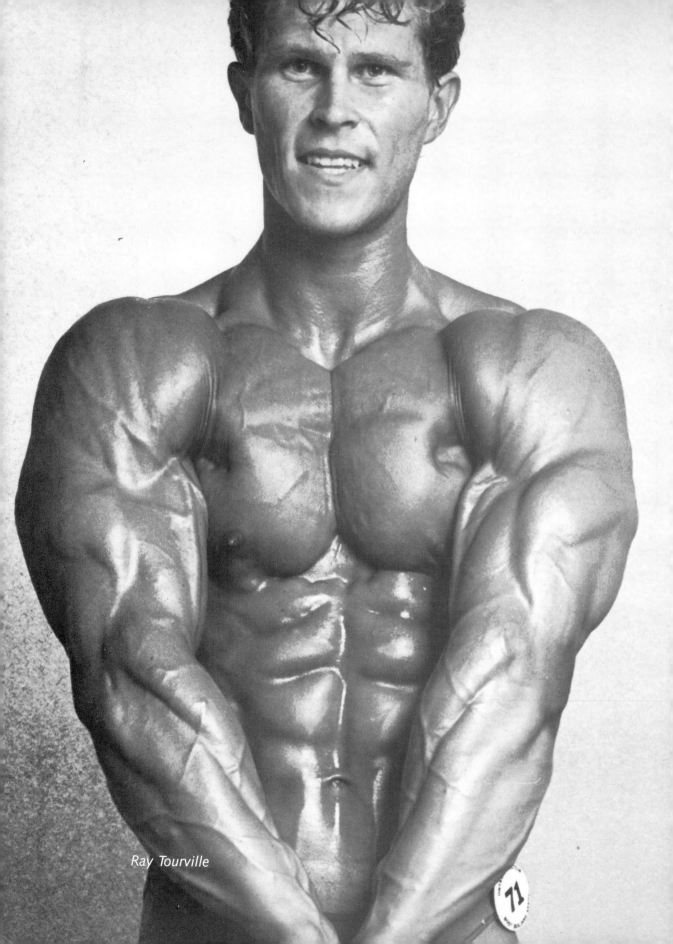

Ray Tourville

71

Stand in front of a full-length mirror and practice tensing each muscle individually. Half a minute will seem like an eternity at first. In time, you will have sufficient control to hold tight for ten minutes at a time—or even more. If you practice enough, the precontest judging will only be mildly exhausting. If you leave everything to the last minute, believing that you will come through when you really need to, then you will curse yourself for not practicing.

The abdominals should be tensed during most of the compulsory front poses, but often this is a matter of personal choice. For example, some bodybuilders like to do a "vacuum" when they do the lat spread or double biceps pose. (For a "vacuum" pose, the bodybuilder inhales deeply and draws in the midsection as tightly as possible.) This is an individual choice you have to make. The question is: Which looks better in your case?

When you are asked to perform the abdominal and thigh poses for the judges, make sure that each official gets a full front view. Pan the judges slowly, looking straight at each judge as you do so. Some competitors like to bend their torsos from side to side to show off their intercostals as well as their abdominal ridges. If you are ripped to shreds, then your intercostals, obliques, and serratus will show up while simply holding a crunched position. It is the man or woman who has a bit too much body fat covering the muscles who should twist and bend. The idea is to prevent a judge from being able to zero in on a weakness.

Flexing the abdominals while posing is not always enough to make the waistline look impressive. You may need to draw your waist in and flex it at the

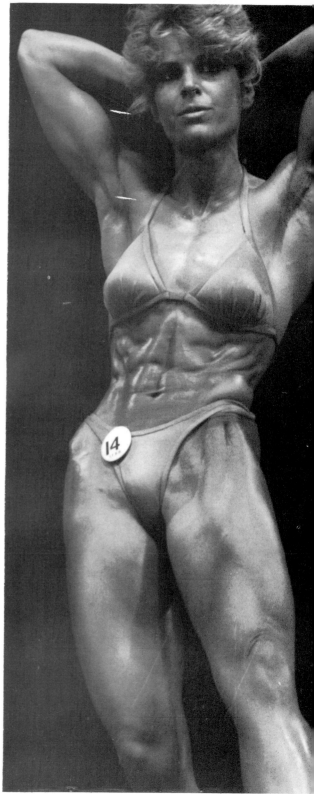

Candy Csencsits

115

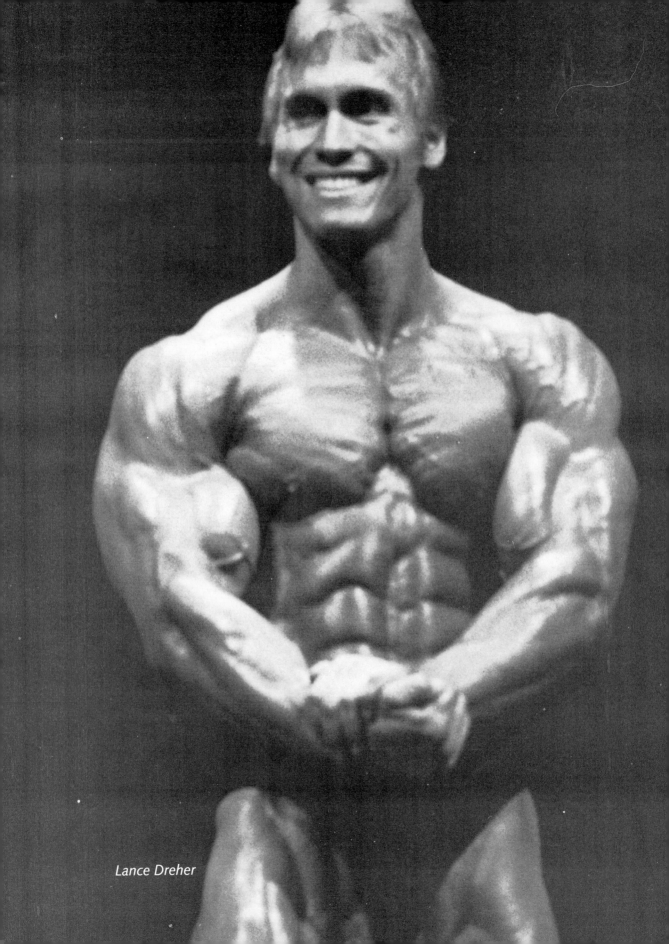

Lance Dreher

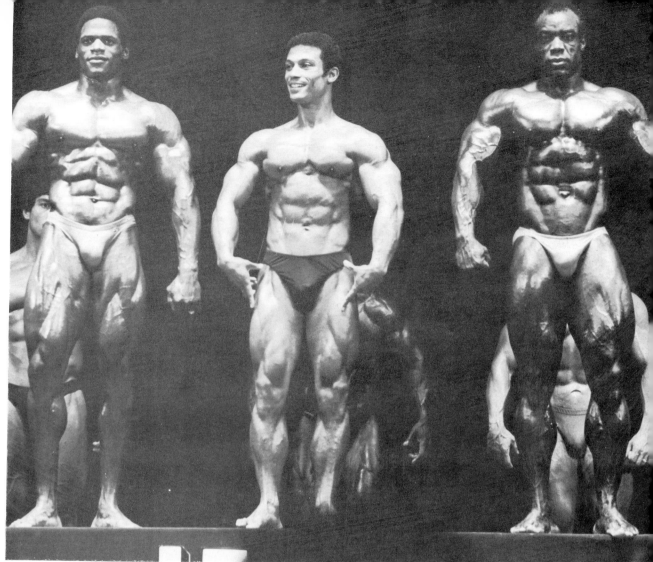

Tony Pearson, Mohamed Makkawy, and Johnny Fuller

same time. In the fifties, most of the competitors were content to merely suck their waists in, to augment the massiveness of the torso. Occasionally, during the relaxed comparisons, you would see one or two abdominal muscles, but for the most part the task was to minimize the waist size. Today, with the increased demands at competitions, it's almost mandatory to draw in the abs *and* flex them.

Today we have a breed of bodybuilders that was unknown in the early years of the sport: bodybuilders with chunky abdominals and bloated waist-

lines. You can blame anabolic steroids for that condition. Taken over a period of time, steroids make almost everything grow, including the intestines. They get fatter and push out your waistline. The *linea alba* (the vertical line between your abdominals) can widen and your once tight abdominals can give the appearance of a swollen pot belly. If you take a lot of steroids, you'll look like a Mack truck. I don't have to tell you which bodybuilders have already done this to their physiques. You only have to look at the pictures. Just don't become one of the gang!

Questions

Gary Leonard and Kay Baxter

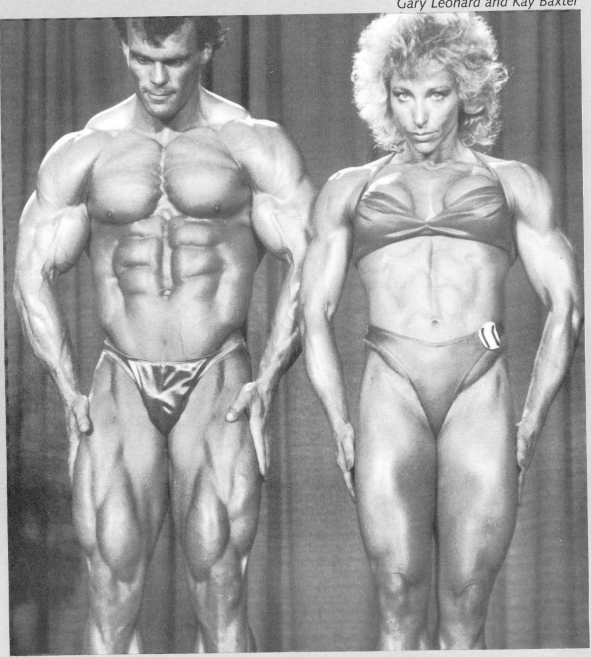

and Answers

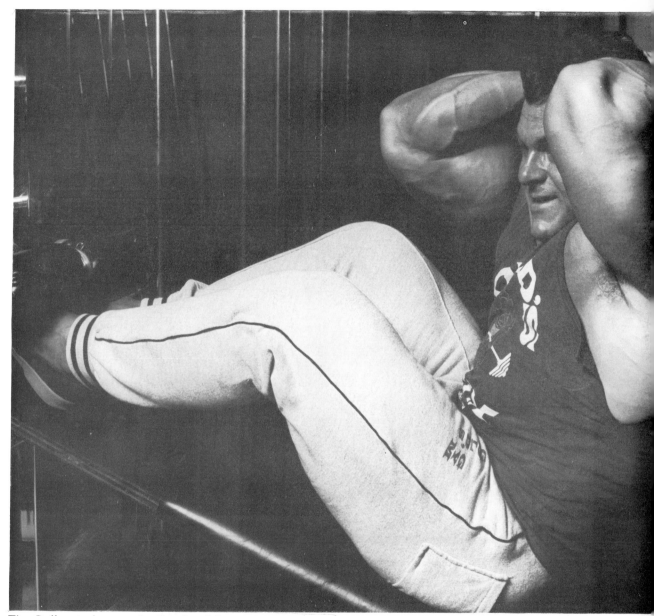

Tim Belknap does an incline bent-knee sit-up.

Question: When I do a crunch or Roman chair sit-up, should I hold my hands behind my head or on my lap?

Answer: Holding your hands behind your head increases the resistance. Placing your hands on your stomach or thighs makes the exercise easier. It all depends on your condition and personal goals. When Arnold Schwarzenegger was training for his Mr. Olympia titles, he would regularly hold his hands behind his head to increase the intensity of the movement. But today, since he doesn't compete in bodybuilding contests anymore, he places his hands on his waist throughout the movement.

Question: I want to add muscle mass to my entire body. How much abdominal exercise should I do?

Answer: Too much ab exercise could throw your body into a kind of nervous shock. As a result, you may find gaining weight difficult. Those interested in gaining mass should limit their abdominal routines to around 10–15 minutes, twice weekly. When you become totally conditioned, you will find that you can work your abs hard with three or four different exercises and still gain muscle mass.

Mike Christian

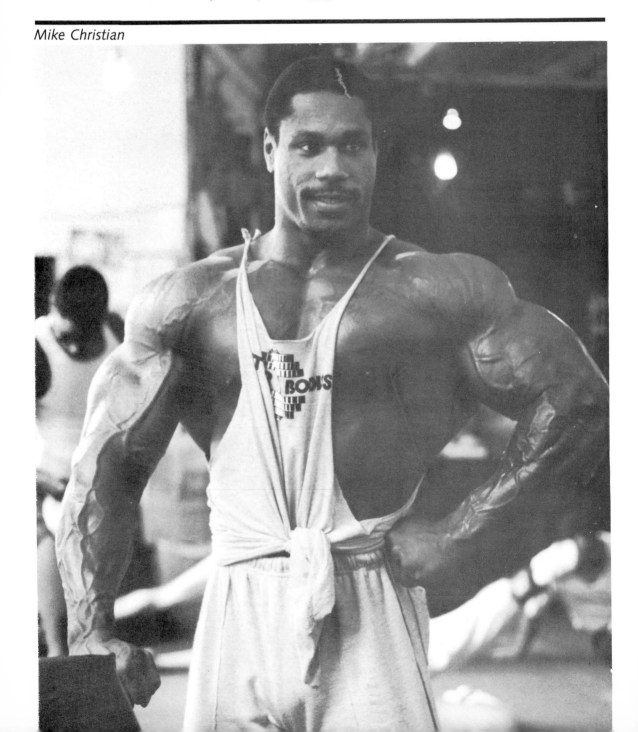

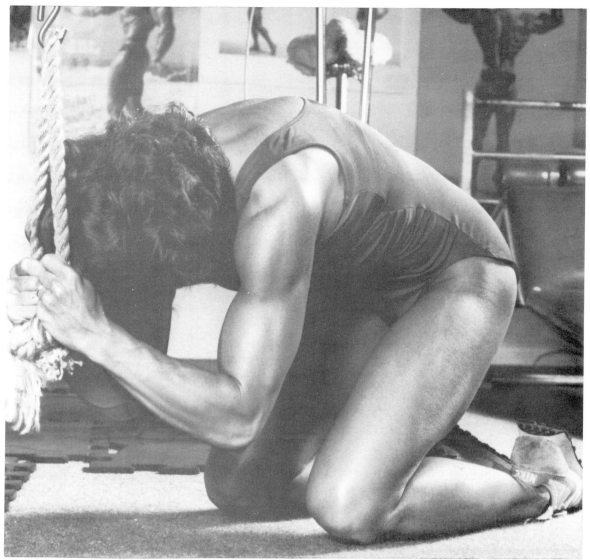

Lynn Conkwright demonstrates an abdominal rope pull.

Question: How should you breathe during abdominal training? I understand that during heavy exercises like squats and bench presses you inhale as the bar or body is lowered and exhale as the most difficult part of the lift is completed. How does breathing work in conjunction with abdominal exercises?

Answer: Because abdominal exercises are often short movements that do not work large muscles of the body, breathing once per repetition is seldom recommended. You just don't need that much oxygen. Try breathing every two or three reps and experiment to determine the best system for each exercise. It is also true that at the beginning of an exercise, for the first reps you will not need to breathe much. However, as the exercise continues and an oxygen debt builds up, you will find yourself breathing with every rep.

Question: I follow Mohamed Makkawy's V.A.T. abdominal-training routine and have made very good progress. Do you advocate this type of training?

Answer: V.A.T. training is short for variable-angle training. Mohamed discovered that parts of each muscle are developed depending on the angle on which the muscle is trained. It is a good idea, especially when training for a contest, to train and develop the muscles from different angles. This makes them pop out with a crystal-clear sharpness, which will gain you extra points during bodybuilding competition.

Mohamed Makkawy does a crunch exercise.

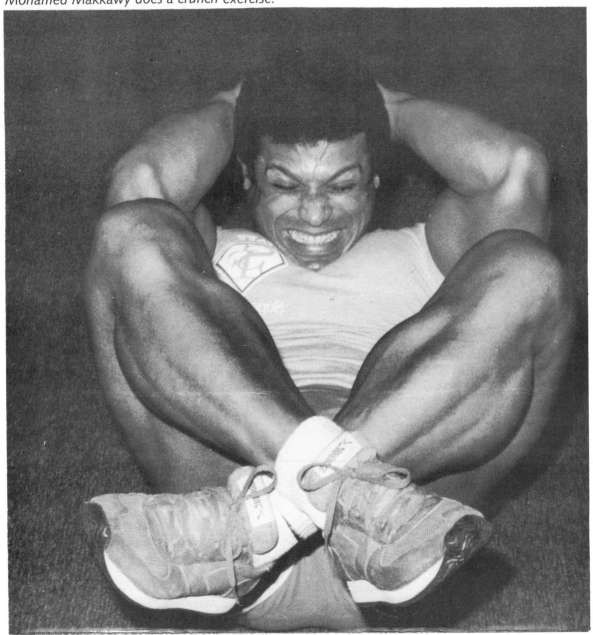

Question: A friend at my gym always does his leg raises, crunches, and Roman chair sit-ups with a twist. Is this a superior method of doing a straight abdominal raise?

Lynne Pirie performs a bench crunch.

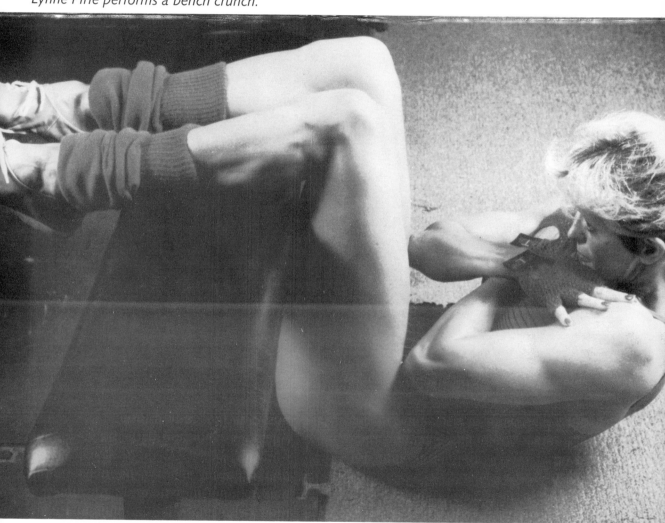

Answer: No. It's a *different* method. I suggest you do straight abdominal work in addition to sets in which twists are used. Then you will be hitting more angles than your friend who *only* does the twisting varieties.

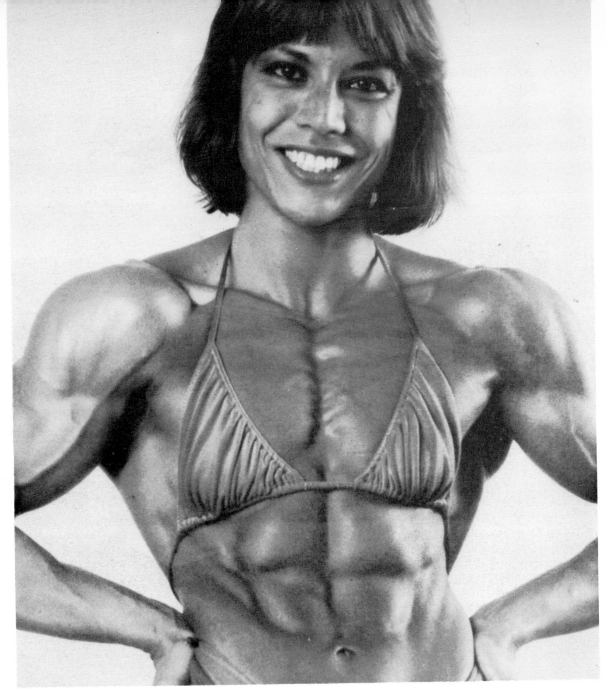

Juliette Bergman

Question: When is the best time to train the abdominals?

Answer: Your abdominal training doesn't usually interfere with the training of any other body parts so you can trim them when you like. Bodybuilders who really want to specialize on their abs may find it advantageous to train them first in a workout, while they are fresh and full of energy. Most people actually leave their ab training to the end of the workout. They find that their dynamic energy is at a lower point, but they still have sufficient energy to give the abs a good training session.

Question: I am genuinely confused over whether I should use additional weight for my abdominal exercises. Should I do more reps with no additional resistance, or should I add weight and do fewer repetitions?

Bertil Fox

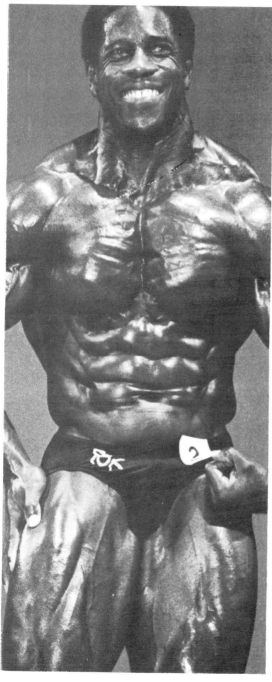

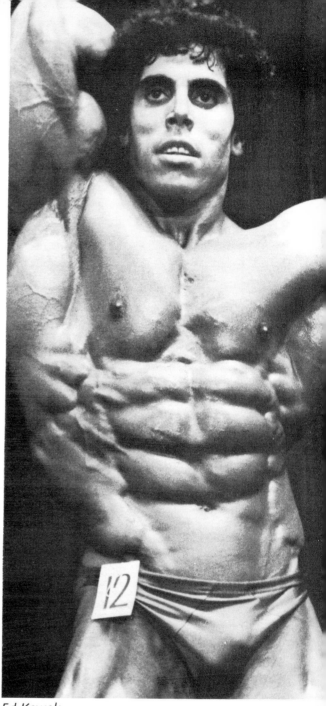

Ed Kawak

Answer: Additional weight will increase the size of your abdominal muscles faster than if you work with higher reps and no weight. Be sure that you are well conditioned before you add extra resistance. Never add weight to a waist exercise before you are able to do scores of reps without added resistance.

Question: Should I train my abs right up to contest time? I usually do my last workout on the Wednesday before a show (if it's on a Saturday). Would it be better if I worked my abs right up to the show date?

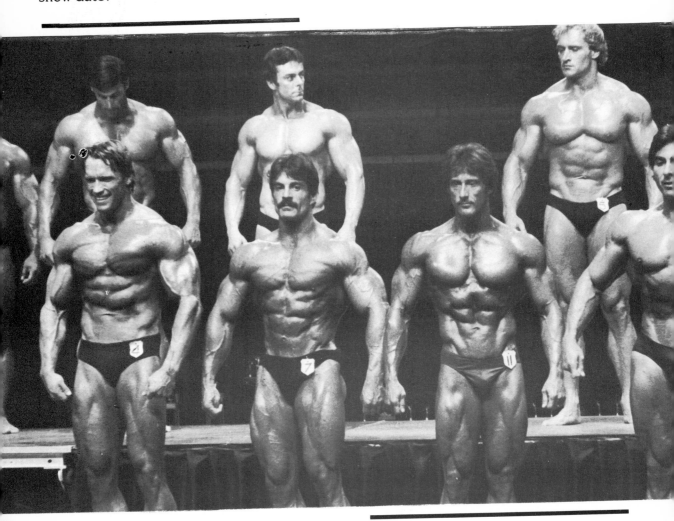

Answer: On the contrary, the abdominals should *not* be exercised at all during the last ten days before a show. Exercising the midsection, as well as improving tone and enlarging muscle size, also increases water retention. Stay away from working those abs before a contest, but keep them maximally toned by regular posing in front of a mirror.

Index